Rock ★ Star MOMMA

★★★★★★★★★★★★★★★★

THE **HIP** GUIDE TO LOOKING **GORGEOUS** THROUGH ALL **NINE MONTHS** AND BEYOND

Skye Hoppus

★

WITH MANDI NORWOOD
& AMY DENOON

ATRIA BOOKS

A Division of Simon & Schuster, Inc.
1230 Avenue of the Americas
New York, NY 10020

First Atria Books paperback edition June 2007

ATRIA BOOKS and colophon are trademarks of Simon & Schuster, Inc.

Interior design by Jaime Putorti
Additional design work by Jennifer Sbranti
Illustrations by Rosemary Fanti Mance

Manufactured in the United States of America

10 9 8 7 6 5 4 3 2 1

Library of Congress Cataloging-in-Publication Data

Hoppus, Skye.
    Rock star momma: the hip guide to looking gorgeous through all nine months and beyond/by Skye Hoppus with Mandi Norwood and Amy Denoon.—1st Atria Books ed.
        p.   cm.
    Includes bibliographical references and index.
    ISBN-13: 978-0-7432-7780-8 (alk. paper)
    ISBN-10:   0-7432-7780-5 (alk. paper)
    1. Pregnancy—Miscellanea. 2. Beauty, Personal. I. Norwood, Mandi.
II. Denoon, Amy. III. Title.

RG525.R6334 2007
618.2—dc22   2006103152

For information about special discounts for bulk purchases, please contact Simon & Schuster Special Sales at 1-800-456-6798 or business@simonandschuster.com.

★ ★

To my family:

Thank you for such a wonderful life.

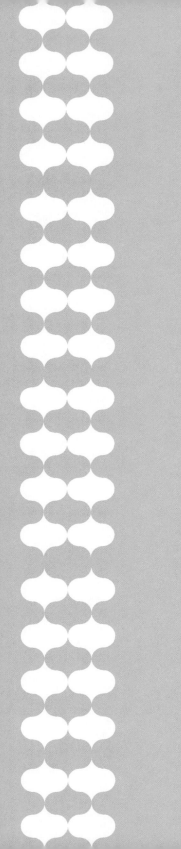

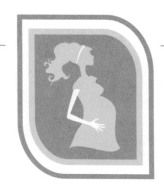

contents

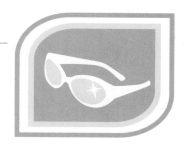

foreword

Being pregnant is an incredible experience in many ways, the physical transformation being the most obvious to the mommy and to the rest of the world. Luckily in our culture, pregnant mommies-to-be can find clothing and ways of dressing that don't totally eradicate our personal style. Most of the time feeling stylish at all is a challenge in and of itself.

Rock Star Momma is full of wonderful ideas and thoughts on putting yourself together that will get you through your pregnancy. The key thing to remember is that this is a time to connect with yourself, be still, go inward, and celebrate the miracle that is your body and the baby that is coming. Feeling pulled together outwardly will do something for you on the days you want to focus a bit on your outside.

Rock Star Momma can help you do that!

—Gwyneth Paltrow

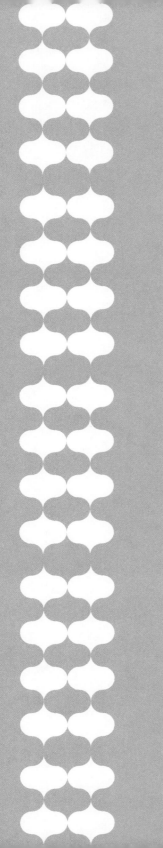

introduction

Congratulations! You're pregnant. Welcome to the club! Now what? Your boobs are sore, you're so tired you can barely make it through the day, and keeping food down has seemingly become an hourly challenge. Your once-perfect complexion? Suddenly your skin is looking like that of an acne-laden teenager, while its hue has taken on a rather pallid, interesting shade of pea green. You're not quite showing yet, but you definitely know that your skinny pants are quickly becoming a thing of the past. Yet you're not sure if you're ready for maternity pants, especially because you remember hearing a secret rule about not wearing them during your first trimester. This is what you signed up for? Never fear, pregnant friend! Soon enough, the cocoon you are bearing will shed way and you will morph into a beautiful, sexy momma-to-be with a gorgeously growing bump.

As you make your glorious transformation from those first few weeks of hormonal upheaval right through to that moment of sheer baby bliss, *Rock Star Momma* is here to help you look and feel amazing even when your complexion is amuck and you're feeling big as a house.

Allow me to introduce myself . . . Skye Hoppus. I'm a mom, wife, designer, stylist, writer, entrepreneur, and a real-life rock star momma—my husband, Mark Hoppus, is one of the founding members of Blink-182 and +44. My son, Jack, is four years old, so I was right where you are now not too long ago—aching boobs, bloated belly, and all. I am also the founder and designer of a very hip maternity (and baby!) line called Childish Clothing. In fact it was out of necessity and luck that Childish was successfully launched, which led to the creation of this here book. I've spent the last three years researching maternity styles and trends and have been blessed to have worked with so many lovely leading ladies during their pregnancies. And let me tell you, I personally gained over fifty pounds while pregnant, so I know what it feels like to experience such monumental changes in your body!

I'm fortunate to have worked with some incredible women and men in this explosive industry and I've asked them to share their expertise with you. I've also asked some of my favorite celebrity friends, and fashion and beauty gurus to pitch in . . . thus the birth of *Rock Star Momma*. You see—believe it or not—there is no hip girl's guide to modern maternity style out there, yet there are four million women each year in the United States alone having babies. Of those four million, I'm betting that more than a few of you want to look and feel fabulous during the most exciting time of your life.

Never mind the fact that in the last few years, being pregnant has become just plain cool—so why not dress the part? Gwyneth, Angelina, Heidi, Kate, Sarah Jessica, Madonna, Gwen, Reese, Mariska, Liv, Catherine, Katie, Courteney, Britney, Brooke, Denise, Debra, Rachel, and Jennifer (that would be Garner!) have all sparked a serious media obsession with all things baby, as well as a whole new era in maternity fashion. Who can forget the groundbreaking 1991 *Vanity Fair* cover with Demi Moore's pregnant nude portrait by überphotographer Annie Leibovitz . . . was this the launch of the maternity revolution? Thanks to these celeb icons, long gone are the days of tent tops and panel pants that were meant to cover up that budding bump. Meet the new maternity maven: she's a gal who looks and feels sexy, beautiful, smart, and confident with babe on board and she's certainly going to dress it. She is a rock star momma.

"Rock star momma" is an attitude that embraces pregnancy and all of its ups and downs. It's about style, sass, and individuality. It's about taking care of you and your baby, and looking great through your entire pregnancy. Because, let's face it, these are the most important months of your life.

I've created a comprehensive fashion, beauty, and well-being guide for you to help navigate your way through the wonderful world of pregnancy while dishing those ever-so-coveted insider and celebrity fashion and beauty secrets to help you exude panache and confidence. I believe in celebrating your changing body (and so should YOU!).

The pages ahead are loaded with an arsenal of invaluable tips-n-tricks, sidebars, and checklists for looking and feeling your best, all the while creating a style that's all your own. Whether it's running errands, hitting the gym, heading to work, going out for a night on the town, or dressing up for a black-tie wedding, *Rock Star Momma* will give you the insider tools for getting splendid style for any occasion, no matter how many months along you may be. Plus, I'll help you deal with getting that hospital bag packed with what you really need, and looking good after Junior arrives—whether you put on twenty-five pounds or sixty.

So with that, read on, have fun, and be stylish, rock star momma! And most important, may your pregnancy be filled with laughter and love, and remember to savor every moment—it goes by way too fast.

—Skye

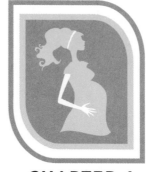

casual *cool*

Whether it's heading to the mall, running errands, grabbing a movie with the girls, or going for a laid-back Sunday morning brunch, "casual cool" is what it's all about. In those pre-pregnancy days, you'd just toss on a tracksuit or an old scrappy T-shirt, some awesome jeans, and a killer belt for instant style. But now that you're knee-deep in hormones and feeling like the human equivalent of a Hummer, getting dressed to run around town isn't the no-brainer it used to be. Even picking out a basic T-shirt can turn into such a daunting task that finding the square root of 126,784,589 seems almost easier. Ah, the joys of hormones, my dear pregnant friend.

Enter Casual Cool. This chapter was created to help make

it easier to achieve relaxed pregnancy style that flatters and feels good, even on those scary, hairy, hormone-laden days. Through the following sections, *Rock Star Momma* will make sure you've got the pregnancy essentials for looks that rock! Check them out:

- ★   Totally Tanks and Tees

- ★   Denim to Die For

- ★   Stellar Skirts

- ★   Terrific Tracksuits

TOTALLY TANKS AND TEES

T-shirts and tank tops are the Holy Grail of casual cool. Whether they're paired with your favorite pair of jeans, comfy trackpants, stylish cargos, or a sassy skirt, tanks and tees are true maternity wardrobe staples. By the very nature of being pregnant, passersby can't help but look at your tummy—and in turn, at that (hopefully) darling tee covering it. So now's the time to step on up and embrace those fun and funky tops like never before. After all, people are looking!

How to find simply fabulous casual cool tees for your belly? It's easy. I promise. First, just say "no!" to those huge, long, tentlike tops. *No, no, no!* Honey, this is the time to delight in your curves, not drown them.

Then, keep in mind the metamorphosis your belly is about to embark upon: from shape and size to how high or low it sits each and every day of your pregnancy. What you'll look for in tops during month three is different from what you'll need by month eight. Thankfully, with the "T-shirts by trimester" guide below, you'll learn all about the hottest tops to wear now through to baby. Read on, maternity maven!

✳ T-SHIRTS BY TRIMESTER

First Trimester

In those early months of pregnancy, even though your bundle of joy is barely the size of a lima bean, your bod is gearing up for the many changes to come and the pounds may be a-packing. You may be feeling so nauseous that the only foods fit to soothe your stomach are laden with comforting but calorie-packed carbs. French fries? Pasta? Cereal? Bagels, anyone? Add hormones to the mix and it's only natural that you may be feeling a little bloated and . . . well, slightly curvier than the pre-pregnancy you. Don't even get me started on the fact that your boobs are about to burst out of your shirt!

That said, it's not quite time for you to make a mad dash to the maternity boutique to outfit your changing shape. If this is your first trip through the wonderful world of pregnancy, you probably won't even "show" until around the seventeenth or eighteenth week—that's over a whole month into your second

first trimester tee tip

Remain calm . . . this is the quiet before the storm. There's really no need yet for real maternity clothes but it sure can be fun looking! Make do with your current wardrobe while you can! I wanted so badly to buy everything right away—and I mean EVERYTHING! Be patient, the time will come soon enough when it's essential to partake in a serious shopping spree. You can always preview the latest fashions on all those great maternity websites out there and build up your wish list so you're prepared when you hit your second trimester. The greatest thing about many of the tees and tanks you probably already have in your wardrobe (aka C&C, Splendid, James Perse, and Juicy, to name a few) is that they all can be worn now as well as transition into your second trimester. You gotta love that comfy cotton jersey that revolutionized the T-shirt market . . . oh, so soft!

trimester. But subsequent pregnancies can start to show between weeks twelve and fifteen.

The best way to conceal that burgeoning bulge during those first few months is to wear tops that flatter and minimize your subtly expanding curves—until, that is, your soft midsection evolves into a firm bump. Boxy and unshapely tees are *never* flattering, but if you are starting to get mushy around the middle, relaxed, languid ones are. Just don't wear your tees so loose that the whole world wonders what you're trying to hide, especially if the nonpregnant you usually sticks to form-fitting shapes . . . you wouldn't want to blow your little secret too soon.

Second Trimester

Sometime during your second trimester your belly is going to pop. And when it does, get ready to have the most fun with your maternity clothes, especially with those tees. But until it does, those first few weeks of the second trimester can be a bit challenging. You know, when you're not big enough to don maternity duds, but you're also just a little too big for your regular clothes?

Rock Star Momma solution: Make friends with s-t-r-e-t-c-h. Cotton or jersey that also contains Lycra or spandex will hug you gently and look sexily slim-fitting, but will grow with you as your belly (and breasts, don't forget) expand.

Second Trimester Tee Tip

It all began one day—almost to the EXACT first day of my second trimester—which I remember as vividly as if it happened this morning, my husband as my witness. That day I headed into my closet and something just felt "different." It was during that time when—and if you haven't experienced this moment yet, then you might want to skip this and come back later!—NOTH-ING, and I mean NOTHING, worked. My belly was getting bigger but not BIG ENOUGH for maternity wear. (Later I realized that this was the moment that drove me to start my own maternity collection.) I wasn't showing enough to convince people I was carrying a child, yet I was far too big to remain looking—and feeling—my normal self. I was knee-deep in that awkward transition time in between showing and not showing and I felt completely and utterly GROSS. Nothing fit. Nothing was comfortable. Nothing looked or felt right. So I did what any hormonal pregnant woman would do: I wept—like a baby!—on my closet floor. After a box of tissues and many reassuring words of comfort from my wonderful husband, I decided to attempt small wardrobe victories one T-shirt at a time. How? I pulled out all my old favorite longer tees and layered them with those stretchy maternity tanks that are so incredibly flatter-ing. I also loved layering a three-quarter-sleeve henley with a con-trasting colored tank. Your husband's Hanes tanks will also come in handy but I say, if you can, splurge for the good maternity styles with added Lycra and length.

POP, THEN SHOP

When you do finally pop, you'll be MORE than ready to shop till you drop! When you head out on your spree, use your pre-pregnancy sizing as a general maternity fit guide, keeping in mind that there isn't a whole lot of consistency in sizing among maternity designers. You may be an extra-small in one brand's tees, but large in another's. Your best bet: Spend some time in the fitting room to assess what works for you. A great maternity store should also have those "fake" bellies that you can Velcro around your existing "new" belly so you can see if that shirt you have your eye on will fit in month nine! Those strap-on bellies (yep, strap-on!) are very useful and hey, it's a fun thing to visualize what's to come while attempting to master your first real maternity wardrobe purchase. Just do it . . . you'll thank me later!

Once you actually LOOK pregnant, don't be afraid to take risks—you can certainly pull it off, maternity momma! Go for fitted tops in bold colors, fun prints, and flattering cuts to create looks that are cool, hip, and totally you. Stick with body-hugging shapes. Why? Because a great fit will accentuate your bump . . . which will then—hooray!—create the illusion of a more slender you everywhere else.

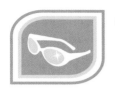

Star Style: Joely Fisher

"There is no way to compare the magnitude, the wonder, the amazement, and humility of being with child, knocked up, having a bun in the oven. It is difficult to describe the unparalleled power in housing another's soul. It's also a bitch to find something to wear. In my chosen profession, I have found that I have had the unfortunate reality of my pregnancies not only having three trimesters, but second halves. The first four or five months is about hiding or masking the 'bump' from the immediate world; therefore, finding a look that is hot and being Houdini (although I hear straightjackets are making a comeback!). It's not that I have found myself unhappy with the bulging belly, just working a little harder at having that sex goddess look I've tried desperately to achieve! Second, only because it works that way—the great reveal, the announcement of the impending addition to our planet. It is at this time that you want to do a naked photo shoot, you are constantly massaging the lump, and you can really belly dance."

—Joely Fisher, actress and mom of two

all shirred up

Shirring is the new pleat—except unlike pleating, it's super-flattering on all body types and is stylishly sexy. No matter what your body, everyone looks great in tops with side or middle shirring. An added plus: shirred fabrics often wrinkle less than other material, ideal for days when you're out and about for hours on end.

Third Trimester

As you work your way toward delivery day, that baby's a-growing at the speed of light, and your belly and boobs look like they're about to burst. So finding great tees and tanks to fit, flatter, and feel great in during those last few months can be HELL.

borrow from the boys

When your belly gets so big that your tees wriggle over your navel and up to your nipples, it's time to steal from your sweetie. Not jackets or shirts—no thanks, he can keep those. I'm talking men's tanks and tees (from the Gap or J. Crew) in sizes XS or small, so they fit sexy and snug across the shoulders but are cut longer in the torso. They make perfect layering pieces for you nearly due mommas!

ear this!

The beauty of tanks and tees lies in their simplicity, right? But casual cool gets serious cred when you wear basics with bold accessories, like drop-dead-gorgeous earrings. As your pregnancy progresses, and your boobs swell to the size of two cantaloupes (and they will), you might want to draw attention away from the obvious. I love the simplicity of a white tank paired with some divine drop or chandelier earrings. So chic!

Here's the key to feeling heavenly again: layering. This little trick will continue to work all the way to birth day. You may think it would add extra bulk, but hold it there! Imagine a fitted, brightly colored camisole in a thin fabric as your bottom layer. Now add a slightly shorter tank top over that (like the cheapie Hanes tank I was talking about), so that the colored cami peaks out from below. Then finish the look with a shorter, long-sleeved, fitted maternity tee. Result? A miraculously elongating (read: *slimming*) effect for your arms and bod, with a look that's fun and funky, too.

☀ BE AWESOME ANYTIME

Besides these must-have trimester tips, this section's got an arsenal of tips that will help you look and feel tee-rific anytime—whether you're in that first, second, or third trimester.

Color Therapy: When you're feeling tired or nauseous, choose bright, colorful tees in colors like hot pink, aqua, apple green, or eggplant. They'll add sparkle back into your complexion, making you look rested and ready for the world (even if you've been up most of the night with an endless urge to pee).

Accentuate Your Assets: Got biceps? If you've got 'em, flaunt 'em, girl! Show them off in a great sleeveless tank. If you've suddenly got boobs, flaunt them with a sexy V-neck or scoop-neck tee.

It's All in the Neck: Necklines are an easy way to change your entire daytime vibe. A basic black tee can be brilliant in a boatneck, sexy in a scoop neck, and dramatic in a drape neck. From a less-is-more crew neck to a va-va-va-voom V-neck, you can completely transform the feel of your outfit by simply switching up your neckline.

Cool and Kitschy: When you're going about your normal non-pregnancy life, the last thing you may ever think about wearing is one of those T-shirts with some kind of corny saying. You know the ones: "J'adore Logos," "You're Fired!" or "Mrs. Pitt." They're just so NOT hot. Yet when you become pregnant, suddenly it becomes more than okay to sport them. That's right—bring on those tees that scream "Baby On Board!" "Got Milk?" "9 Months," "Breeder," and, of course, "Rock Star Momma"! You're clearly pregnant, so why not have some fun with these clever shirts that humorously declare your pregnancy to the world? You'll pretty much never be able to wear them again, so go for it.

Support to a Tee: Feel the need for extra control up top now that your boobs are bigger? You can still achieve casual cool in tees that come with a built-in bra, offering additional support to your two new, fuller friends. (They'll give extra camouflage to darkening nipples, too.)

Casual and Comfortable: As skin stretches, it becomes itchy and sensitive. Don't add to the trauma with synthetics. Choose tees and tanks in tissue-soft cottons and jerseys

buff biceps

It's really important to stay fit during your entire pregnancy by exercising. Working out every day is good for you and Junior, too. In fact, exercising even before you're pregnant has been shown to improve the way you'll feel in your icky, sicky, exhausting first trimester. And according to the American Academy of Family Physicians, women who keep fit throughout their entire pregnancies have healthier, easier, shorter labors than women who don't. *(Of course, you must chat with your doctor about all this before you hit the gym.)* But there are other bonuses, too—such as looking better. The very best pregnancy exercise of all is swimming. Not only are you giving your body a superb aerobic workout (good for your heart and lungs), it's the best way to strengthen and tone your arms and legs. So you'll look hot in a T-shirt or tank, and most important, when your beautiful babe arrives, those biceps will be ready for all the lifting that comes with a newborn. And believe me, those infant carriers get *heavy*.

FROM A PRO

"Pair a novelty tee with your favorite pair of jeans for a look that can easily change with your mood. These fun and funky tees are the perfect way to make your maternity wardrobe hip yet comfortable at the same time."

—SHANNON DiPADOVA,
founder of Due Maternity boutiques and website

(cashmere is also nice if the weather—and your wallet!—allows), natural, breathable fabrics that stretch, soothe the skin, and keep you casually cool even when it's ninety degrees and rising.

Simply Sleeves: Whether it's due to weight gain, water retention, or both, many women complain that their arms magically expand during pregnancy. The solution? Get creative with your sleeves to create a look that flatters all shapes and sizes:

✓ **Get Shorty:** Contrary to popular belief, cap sleeves are always great. They open up your shoulders, making your waist and arms appear smaller, which is an especially handy trick during those last few months.

✓ **Three-quarter:** You can't go wrong here. No matter what size your arms may be, three-quarter sleeves give coverage where you need it, yet offer just the right amount of sexiness and sass. Try fitted sleeves for a more sporty vibe or a looser, free-flow arm for a more romantic look.

✓ **Long and Lovely:** Long sleeves suit you best? Looking for a top that also takes you to work? A bell sleeve or a gentle flare is great for hiding heavy upper arms and adds a touch of whimsy to any look.

REVOLUTIONIZING MATERNITY FASHION

"We believe that just because you're pregnant, it doesn't mean you have to lose your sense of style. It's all about comfort, style, and sexy clothes that make you feel great all through your pregnancy—and after. Whether you're a mom-to-be in your twenties, thirties, or forties, you want comfort, you want style, and you definitely want to stay looking good throughout your entire pregnancy. Versatile pieces are key to building a great maternity wardrobe at any age, giving you multiple looks and options, without you having to invest too much in clothing you can only wear for a few months. In your twenties, skirts can be thrown on with flip-flops and a tank or dressed up with heels and a sexy top to go from work to weekend. In your thirties, curve-hugging dresses will do the same, giving you the option to wear them out to dinner or as a beach cover-up. More tailored pieces, like collared shirts and flat-front pants, look great if you're in your forties, allowing you to look chic and pulled together with a sophisticated touch."

—LAURIE McCARTNEY,
founder of babystyle

⊘ T-SHIRT NO-NO'S

So there you have it—Tees and Tanks 101 to help you get through any month of your pregnancy in comfort and style. Just one last thing before moving on to Denim to Die For. While I know that you'd never be guilty of committing the following tanks and tees no-no's, I just need to list them for my own little peace of mind. Don't fall victim to any of these fashion faux pas, no matter what your hormones are telling you:

- ✗   Too tight is never just right. If you can't breathe when you get it on—or you can see bra-strap bulge—it's time to part ways. Bra-strap bulge is NEVER sexy!

- ✗   Vintage is cool . . . dirty, tattered, and falling apart is NOT!

- ✗   Forgo horizontal stripes. Diagonal and vertical are fine, but you're already on your way to getting big, so don't do anything that might make you look bigger, okay?

DENIM TO DIE FOR

Thanks to the advent of those famous 501s a hundred and fifty years ago, jeans are a major part of our daily twenty-first-century wardrobe—whether it's to the office, for a night out on the town, or running those endless errands. Yet considering how often you wear them, it's still shocking at how hard it is to find the perfect pair. Now try adding pregnancy and a whole lotta pounds to the equation. Yikes! Don't fret. Why? Because you're gonna make your first major maternity investment right now. (Pause for effect.) You. Are. Going. To. Buy. A. Pair. Of. Maternity. Jeans.

I know, I know. I understand you're glued to your Sevens and Hudsons. I know it's terrifying to imagine life without your Citizens or True Religions. But take a deep breath and listen to me: Your behind is going to get bigger. Your hips, legs, and thighs, too. And you've probably already lost that thing you once so proudly called your "waist." Maternity jeans are designed with all these things in mind—unlike regular jeans, which are designed for supermodels (which explains why finding the perfect fit for mortals is so insanely difficult).

Truth is, maternity jeans have come a very long way from what they were even a few years ago. Phew. Whereas once upon a

FROM A PRO

"Invest in a great pair of jeans, they are more than worth it! Denim is the hottest trend out there and will continue to be. Just like your nonprego jeans, you will wear them constantly. Splurge on a pair that makes you look and feel gorgeous!"

—SHANNON DiPADOVA,
founder of Due Maternity boutiques and website

FROM A PRO

"Designer denim . . . they are HOT in ready to wear so they are HOT in maternity. Today's denim is worn so fitted. It's generally the first item of staple clothing pregnant women buy. And nothing makes a butt look better than a great pair of designer jeans!"

—SONG PARDUE,
CEO, Pickles and Ice Cream, key retailer

time, maternity jeans were those full-paneled "mom jeans"—with a panel so high, it could readily be mistaken for some sort of breast support, and those giant, unflattering pockets made even Twiggy's ass look the size of Texas—today's pregnancy jeans are available in a plethora of hip styles that'll make even the most stylish momma smile.

Use your pre-pregnancy sizing as a general reference for maternity sizing, but as with tees, there really isn't much consistency among maternity brands. If you can't bear the thought of those scary dressing room mirrors, order online and try dozens on in the comfort of your own home. But remember: Ignore what the numbers say on the tag and go for what truly fits (repeat the mantra: "I am embracing the new me"). While you're at it, follow the handy guide below to finding the perfect pair of kick-ass maternity jeans.

THE ROCKIN' GUIDE TO ALL THINGS JEANS

★ **Stretch, Baby, Stretch:** Those jeans have just got to have stretch. Think major S-T-R-E-T-C-H, momma, because that's what's going to keep those jeans fitting from month five through your trip to the delivery room. Look for somewhere between two and eight percent Lycra or spandex to ensure that your jeans will grow with you while still keeping their shape. A good pair of maternity jeans should fit fabulously throughout your entire pregnancy!

★ **The Right Rinse:** The general rule of thumb is that the darker the denim rinse, the more slenderizing it is. I say stick with darker washes and avoid lighter ones (especially those ass-enlarging acid washes of the eighties). If you're trying to conceal a particular area, steer clear of distressing in that given spot. For instance, if you've got largish thighs already, don't wear jeans that have distressing at the tops of the legs. Get it?

★ **Fab Fabric:** Comfort is SO key during your pregnancy, especially when it comes to your jeans. Go for soft, washed denims, rather than superstiff, heavy jeans. I'm loving the new "jeano"—a buttery-soft cross between jeans and chino that you can wear for hours and still feel great. And rumor has it, supersmart, momma-friendly designers are working with cashmere-denim blends. The gods have answered!

★ **Perfect Pockets:** Ah, the endless quest for those perfectly placed booty pockets—you know, the ones that'll miraculously lift, shrink, and shape all in one? Here's the inside secret to finding them (they DO exist!): Choose jeans with larger back pockets that are pro-

new classics

The denim market has been on fire and there's no sign of it slowing down! Be sure to check out the latest round of new classics in denim:

- Deep indigos and straight legs are definitely making waves!
- Devilshly dark and ultra-skinny style rocks! That is, only if you've got legs like those ZZ Top sings about!
- Super-soft enzyme-washed denim in fresh tones of ocean blue

fashion tip

If you're on the shorter side, try a longer cut with a great pair of heeled boots or shoes. An espadrille wedge sandal—in gold, platinum, or bronze—adds leg length and glamour.

portionally placed in the center of each cheek. If they're placed too high up or are too small in size, they'll make your butt look bigger. If you opt for pocketless denim, go for jeans that have a deep V yoke at the back to create the illusion of "cleavage."

★ **She's Got Legs:** From boot-cut to loose leg . . . no matter what kind of style you choose, one thing should always be consistent: longer equals leaner. Boot-leg and gentle-flare cuts look great on every bod—no matter how tall, short, big, or small you may be. If you're tall and slender, you can pull off a wide-leg cut, too.

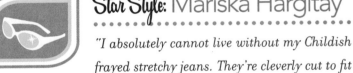

Star Style: Mariska Hargitay

"I absolutely cannot live without my Childish frayed stretchy jeans. They're cleverly cut to fit below the belly, yet they never migrate downward or make me look like a plumber. Plus, they really talk to a pregnant chick . . . their tag says, 'You Are Beautiful . . . Rock On!'"

—*Mariska Hargitay,* actress and mom

★ **Waist-land:** There are so many different options for waistbands these days, but my favorite is consistently a soft under-the-belly waistband. It's the only one that's truly comfortable from sunrise to sundown and works great all the way through to delivery and into postpartum. Some have a gentle supportive waistband, while others just offer a lot of stretch around the waist—to give the illusion of nonmaternity jeans—and are ideal for days when you want to wear those shorter, fitted tees and tanks.

★ **Last Resort:** If you just can't be separated from your Blue Cults or Paige Premiums, think about customizing them into your own special maternity jeans. You can buy maternity panels from sewing or notions stores and ask a tailor to sew them into your favorite pair. Voilà!

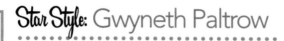

Star Style: Gwyneth Paltrow

"I preferred simple clothing myself, on a daily basis, and I found it relatively easy to find things to wear. Stretchy jeans and T-shirt dresses, lots of layering and cardigans. I think the thing to remember when you are pregnant is comfort and ease. Sometimes just your hair scraped back with some nice earrings are enough to spruce up the jeans and shirt that you wear every day. And accessories are a great way to feel a bit stylish."

—*Gwyneth Paltrow,* actress and mom

❋ The Quick-n-Dirty

Wanna find the best jean for your bod? Read on . . .

IF YOU ARE:	THEN TRY:
Heavy around the tushie	Boot-cut with wide back pockets set high and close to the center to minimize a wide butt; if they're too small, that booty will look even bigger. Avoid distressing around the butt—it'll only call attention to your derriere.
Heavy thighs	A long boot-cut or straight (not narrow) leg is superslimming. Look for jeans that are darker at the edges of the legs than at the center, with a whiskered look (whitish "crumple lines" in the inner thigh), which creates a slenderizing illusion. Remember: The shorter the jean, the shorter—and heavier—your legs will look.
Long and lean	Lucky you! Pretty much any style works, but I always love a gentle flare. If you're supertall, look for at least a thirty-five-inch inseam (the average inseam is around thirty-two inches) so it's long enough to graze the top of your shoes in the front and hit halfway between your heel and your ankle in back.
Short and hippy	Stay clear of lighter washes—they make everyone look larger. Instead, opt for a boot or flared leg in a soft, stretchy fabric with a dark or antique rinse—and wear with a pair of sexy stilettos. Need to shorten jeans, but don't want to lose that cool "jeans" hem? Take them to a tailor who has yellow-gold jeans thread. (Tip: If the hems of your freshly shortened jeans look unnaturally clean, run an emery board or cheese grater over them for a distressed finish in seconds!)

Heidi Klum

Now, I must preface this story with the fact that MOST pregnant women are not as genetically blessed with a body and legs like Heidi Klum. Yes, I know you are all probably praying daily to the maternity god to have a body like Heidi had during (all!) her pregnancies. With that said, I received a call one day last year from Heidi, who had fallen in love with my denim pieces but wanted a more fitted style. She wanted "skinny" jeans. Without hesitation, I dashed to the sewing room and created a maternity skinny jean—something I thought I would never do! "Maternity" and "skinny" are just not synonymous but in this case, it felt like two peas in a pod. And, to date, I continue to manufacture this style!

FROM A PRO

"In the past six years since I have been fashion editor for *Fit Pregnancy* magazine, and pregnant with my son, maternity clothes have gotten quite a style makeover. It's no wonder everyone in Hollywood is getting pregnant. They can't wait to wear the amazing maternity clothes available now. If you're going to make one investment while you're pregnant, splurge on a pair of maternity jeans. There are so many to choose from and no one would ever guess they're maternity jeans!"

—KATHRYN McRITCHIE,
fashion editor at *Fit Pregnancy*

✳ JEAN-IOUS ACCESSORIES

Hopefully I've taught you well and by now you've probably got the jeans thing mastered, right? So while you're at it, why not get a little funky and have some serious fun with your denim? If the length allows, cut off a touch at the bottom of the legs, then wash to give it those unfinished edges. Try sewing a patch or two on the front or back pockets, or try aptly positioning vintage silk pins on your front pockets, or add a stunning silk scarf that doubles as a belt . . . all make a serious statement on your jeans and your style. Very Gucci a la 1980! *Wow!*

Star Style: Kimora Lee Simmons

"Baby Phat jeans were my must-have item in my maternity wardrobe because they have so much stretch, more stretch than any other jeans I have tried. I was able to wear them well into my pregnancy instead of having to shop for maternity jeans."

—Kimora Lee Simmons

model, creative director of Baby Phat, and mom

Denim Diary

Some women's friend, some women's enemy, jeans have never really been my best friend; more like an acquaintance. As if it's not hard enough trying to find the perfect jeans on a normal day, as you now probably know, trying to find a great pair of jeans when pregnant can feel like a losing battle. When I was pregnant, there were no "cool" maternity jeans. So I bought those mediocre, paneled (yes, *gross*) maternity jeans and literally tore them up. I took scissors to them—a la Edward Scissorhands style—and went at it! Hey, why not. After all, it made those miserable, drab jeans feel and look like something I would've worn any other day. Create something of your own, a style all your own. You know your limits and what makes you feel and look your best. Simple adjustments with a little flair will do the trick. Trust me, it will make the thought of maternity jeans far more palatable to even the biggest fashion slave. Another piece of advice: Longer is always the way to go. It elongates those legs—and mine needed all the help they could get. I always chose a longer fit and paired them with a sexy stiletto or my favorite chocolate-brown knee-high Prada boots. Sexy, sophisticated, and a look that carried me perfectly from day into night.

⊘ DENIM DON'TS

Whatever route you choose to go, I leave you with a few little "denim don'ts"—you know, things that should just never, ever happen with your jeans. I'm pretty darn sure you'd never go there, but hey, better safe than sorry:

- ✗ Never. Wear. Acid. Washed. Jeans. Ever.

- ✗ Crack just ain't cool (see the **Panty Shmanty** chapter for more on this one, gals), so just don't show it.

- ✗ Ditch jeans (or any trousers, maternity or not, for that matter) with pleats, as they'll only make you look bigger.

- ✗ Avoid the ripple effect; that is, jeans that create a ripple on your inner thighs. This is a clear indicator that your pants don't fit, so size up and/or look for a different style.

- ✗ Tapered jeans are *never* cool.

- ✗ Don't resort to your husband's jeans. They may feel comfortable, but they'll do nothing for your butt . . . even if you do cinch the waist with a Roberto Cavalli belt.

- ✗ Don't be seen in the Texas tuxedo—a denim jeans and denim jacket together. Just not chic. If you can't be persuaded, at least wear a light-hued jacket with dark-hued jeans. But please, puh-leeze, avoid light and light—we love him, but you don't really want to look like Jon Bon Jovi circa *Slippery When Wet*.

✗   Need I even bother to say this? Denim overalls are meant to stay on the farm, not in your wardrobe—not now, not ever!

STELLAR SKIRTS

Sometimes pants just won't do. Like when it's midsummer and it's so hot outside, your legs have swollen and the very idea of stuffing them into pants causes your heart rate to soar. Or in spring when you're feeling light and airy and you want to celebrate your femininity as you're out tackling the town. Perhaps it's in the dead of winter when a mini, some bright tights, and knee-high boots call to your inner fashion goddess. Sometimes a great skirt is just what the doctor ordered for creating casual cool. Whether you're at month four or month eight, here's how to look simply stellar in skirts:

Star Style: Joely Fisher

"Fortunately for us Gen-Xers, pregnancy doesn't mean the end of style, sensuality, and sexiness—my 'maternity' look didn't stray far from my skinny-bitch look. I shopped in two maternity stores and then stayed with my regular haunts. . . . I sashayed my way through twenty glorious months and I have two gorgeous girl-flavored children to prove it. Now back to the crunches!"

THE SIMPLY STELLAR GUIDE TO ALL THINGS SKIRTS

Mini Madness: There's just something to be said about a great mini. It's a little bit sweet, a little bit sexy, and all parts chic. Whether it's ruffled terry or daring denim, miniskirts are pure magic for rock star mommas. Supercurvy or hippy gals: Look for slightly longer minis, so that any trouble spots are well hidden. Whatever your size, use your best judgment when it comes to length—that behind should always be well covered.

Amazing A-line: No matter what your body type—from straight and skinny to completely curvy—A-line skirts flatter all. They shrink hips if you've got 'em, while creating flattering curves on a straight frame. Tip: Best worn until month seven, when your belly will be so big, you'll start to look like a ship in full sail.

Wrap Skirts: Gotta love the wrap skirt. This staple is ideal for every stage of pregnancy, especially if you feel really comfortable with a low, under-the-belly waist. The beauty of this skirt is that you can wrap it as loose or as tight as you want, so it can grow with you through your pregnancy. Make them your belly's best friend in any color or print—from neutral tones and bright colors to funky patterns and asymmetrical edges.

Pencil Skirts: Show off that new booty and those sexy hips in a pencil skirt! Paired with your favorite tee and casual shoes, a pencil skirt immediately imparts subtle sophistication into your everyday look. Or, elongate your frame by tossing on a pair of peep-toe heels. Note to self: Fit is key here and if there is EVER any doubt as to whether you can pull this off, then refrain and try something more appropriate for your body.

Long and Lovely: When opting for long skirts, think really, really long . . . as in just about grazing the floor—if your skirt hits in between your calves and the top of your shoes, you risk looking shorter and . . . well, rounder. Try layered or tiered long skirts to add a touch of bohemian beauty to any casual look. When going long and lovely, it's best if you wear flats or sandals. The cool factor completely disappears when paired with heels.

stellar skirt style

Are spider veins starting to creep up on your legs and scaring you from wearing skirts? Ah, just one more joyous perk of pregnancy. How to cover? In the winter, opt for dark-colored tights and in the summer, use body bronzers and doctor-approved self-tanners. Another way to funk it up . . . go for fishnets, baby (if you dare!). They'll add a little flair while disguising those heinous veins.

THE QUICK-N-DIRTY GUIDE TO SKIRTS THAT SCREAM "HOT MOMMA"

When done right, skirts are a rockin' part of your maternity wardrobe through all nine months. The following is a quickie skirt-style checklist to make sure you've got all the basics covered:

The right length	When in doubt, the best length for all body types is just below the knee, hitting at the narrowest part of the leg.
Big booty	A-line, gentle tiering, or layers are best to help diminish that derriere.
No booty	Look for flattering back pockets, yoking, or ruffles to add bulk where there is none. And an A-line will give the effect of more!
Short	Pencil skirts that hit just below the knee. Look for vertical detailing (pinstripes or waist-to-hem stitching) to elongate you.
Tall	Anything goes—just make sure that if it's short, your tushie is covered, and if it's long, that it grazes the floor.

a-hem! which heels to wear

The wrong shoe can take the wow out of the most wonderful skirt. Here are your shoe and skirt solutions:

SKIRT	SHOE
Mini	Flats, slides, thongs. No heels, unless you're Heidi Klum
Pencil	Heels—two and a half inches—make a commanding partner; knee-high wickedly soft and supple leather boots are HOT
A-line	Delicate kitten heels slenderize (or thongs in the summer months)
Mid-length tiered	Stacked or wedge heels help balance skirt shape—or for you thinner gals, thongs will work, too
Ankle-length	Flats, jeweled or metallic thongs, or ballet flats

Ø SKIRT NO-NO'S

So there you have it. See? Skirts are actually surprisingly simple during pregnancy. A few last thoughts to make sure your skirt style is always stunning:

✘ A skirt that hits at your midcalf (usually the biggest part of your lower leg) is never, ever flattering.

✘ I see London. I see France. I see pregnant

chickie's underpants. Whether it's how you sit or how you bend over, just make sure it doesn't happen. Crack ain't cool . . . especially now!

✘ Pleats are never pretty. They just make you look bigger and boxier.

✘ Bulky, heavy fabrics will make you look just that: bulkier and heavier.

FROM A PRO

"Maternity clothing has changed so radically in the past few years that I can honestly say that most women I get my hands on actually look hipper and more stylish than in their non-maternity wardrobe. They are more willing to take chances, happy to show some newfound cleavage, and for the most part actually feel sexier."
—DEBBIE OHANIAN,
   designer and founder of Meet Me in Miami

TERRIFIC TRACKSUITS

Just a few years ago, the thought of a hip girl wearing a track-suit—other than to the gym—was just plain nuts. Rather, upon hearing the very word, an immediate flood of childhood memories could easily be evoked: Senior citizens heading to Denny's. John Travolta in *Perfect*. Old-school Run-DMC in Fila. Nope, tracksuits certainly weren't must-haves for the fashionably hip, least of all rock star mommas.

But then, something big happened. Something really big and . . . well . . . juicy. Juicy Couture helped make tracksuits cool with their flattering cuts, comfortable fabrics, and sexy feel. Within no time, tracksuit couture became synonymous with serious style and other designers quickly followed suit. Trendsetting stars like Madonna and Jennifer Lopez warmly embraced the trend, establishing its place in our culture and prompting millions of women to buy into the wardrobe staple.

During pregnancy, tracksuits come in handier than ever. From running errands to hitting the gym, donning stretchy, below-the-belly waistband trackpants in breathable fabrics worn with a fitted tee is an instant way to add major style and comfort to any maternity wardrobe. Whether it's bright and bold, long and loose, or cropped and comfy, track-suits are the way to go. Plus, not only do they make a stylin' outfit on their own, split up and paired with other pieces—like

DID YOU KNOW?

. . . That Juicy Couture actually started out as Travis Jeans, a line of maternity jeans named after founder Gela Nash-Taylor's son Travis?

a sexy tank with trackpants, a zip-up hoodie with a flirty skirt—tracksuits can provide endless casual cool options.

Postpartum, tracksuits are the perfect solution to looking cute while hiding those trouble spots that we all develop during pregnancy. Functionally, a zip-up hoodie makes breastfeeding a breeze, while the stretchy waistband on trackpants lets you be comfortable at any time—whether it's for those endless hours of feeding, burping, and changing or for doing one of those yoga videos that keep calling your name!

baby's got bling!

Pregnancy is your time to make a brilliantly bold statement with accessories. Tossing on a trendy pair of big earrings or a fun scarf with your tracksuit is an easy way to add sass and style, while drawing attention to your face—and away from your growing belly and booty.

color blind

Go ahead and add some color with your bag. Experiment with provocative hues, but be sure they don't compete with what you're wearing. Pick a shade that is bold yet pretty, and one that complements your wardrobe. And girls, remember, the days of matchy-match style are *long gone*!!

Swipe Her Style: Brooke Shields

Being casual cool during your pregnancy never looked so good! Brooke Shields made it look so easy and just plain cool. I just love how she pulled together her look. Exuding confidence, style, and personality, she paired a bucket hat with a navy velour tracksuit to add a touch of individuality for a terrific look. To find out how you can acheive this look, refer to Brooke's illustration in the **Swipe Their Style** *chapter.*

Tracksuit Trimester Checklist

Have fun and take some risks, but be sure to keep in mind these few basic style tips to keep you looking your best in tracksuits.

FIRST TRIMESTER

✓ Look for a looser fit that's all about comfort. Since you may not be feeling so great during those first twelve weeks (nausea and exhaustion, anyone?), the focus should be on wearing clothes that are so comfortable—and cute—that they can't help but make you feel better.

✓ Bright, cheery colors will help your skin escape the pallid hue that you just might be experiencing.

✓ Wide waistbands will ensure your tracksuit's the perfect retreat when your tummy needs relief from increasingly tight clothes.

SECOND TRIMESTER

✓ Look for jackets that have a longer torso, so that as you grow, your jacket will keep its fit.

✓ Pants with stretchy, low elastic waists are most flattering on all body types and heights. Look for lots of Lycra or spandex in the band's content for added support and comfort.

THIRD TRIMESTER

✓ Think big. Think sexy. Wearing a tracksuit that barely covers your tummy is a subtle way to add a little sex appeal—especially in your last trimester when that bump is supersized—and to show that belly off to the world!

✓ Getting really, really big? As in "even my biggest pregnancy clothes are starting not to fit"? Just toss on your track jacket and wear it open over a simple tank top or two. This look is especially cute when you layer your tanks—think white Hanes racerback tanks (like six bucks at Kmart)—which go a long, long way no matter how big you are.

Riding in Buses with Belly

Imagine this: Seven months pregnant, a tour bus, hot summer days, long drives, swollen ankles . . . not the ideal combination, right? Well, all's fair in the name of love and devotion. Not your typical vision of backstage at a rock show? Thanks to the many terry tracksuits I traveled with and a load of old comfy tees, I managed to make it, and make it in a style all my own. The key for me was to have the basic hoodie and drawstring trackpants that accentuated those newfound curves, yet managed to hide those "flaws." You know what I mean, girls!

The key is to choose pieces that are flattering to show off your belly, not hide it. Steer clear of overly loose, big tops and bottoms to avoid looking heavy instead of hot. Also, get creative—make a simple tank top a classic by adding your own personal embellishments. Ribbons for a little girlish flair, vintage pins for a spark of class, or sew on an old Rolling Stones patch you still have saved in your closet. It's fun, easy, and, most important, you!

❋ ANYTIME TRACKSUIT TIPS

Loose and Low: Wear those pants loose and low on your hips—it is simply slimming for all body types. (Just watch out for panty peek-a-boos—you don't want your pants so low that you cross the thin line between cute and crude!)

Bigger Is Sometimes Better: If you try on a tracksuit that just fits, consider buying a size up to help get the most wear for your buck. And remember that if the tracksuit has any Lycra in the content, then you can be pretty sure that your suit will shrink . . . so be safe and bump—no pun intended—up a size.

Cropped Can Be Cute: That is, as long as those ankles haven't turned to cankles (you know, when your calves and ankles mesh into one), which is common when you're retaining water toward the end of your pregnancy. If you do go for cropped, they look best with thongs or sneakers. If you wear socks with your sneakers, be sure to wear ankle socks. Want some WOW? Try sparkly gold rhinestone thongs, toss on some big chunky earrings, add a cute scarf, and wear a sexy tank underneath. Voilà!

Color Me Bright: Think bright, bold, and brilliant. Mix 'em up with colorful combos. Hot pink, army green, and camouflage are all superstylish ways to go.

Old School: Wear a vintage tee or tank under any tracksuit for anytime cool. Thrift-store tees can be groovy, unique, and so comfortable!

tracksuit tresses

Whether you're off to yoga or heading out for a shopping spree, you'll need a tame mane to pull off tracksuit trendy with panache. Help prevent unwanted frizzies and fly-aways by using a weightless, strong-hold styling product—such as Aveda Self Control Hair Styling Stick—on the ends after blow-drying and, if needed, at your hair line to smooth down unruly strays. Spritz on a little shine spray for some extra luminosity and vibrance. For the ultimate in modern, sexy, casual hair, wear it stick straight, in a pony, or soft and wavy.

Fabric Finds: When it comes to tracksuits, have fun with fabrics—no matter what your size. Whether it's terry, velour, or thermal, they all work. And again, cashmere is always a luxury!

the last word

⭐ It's hard to go wrong with tracksuits—they're just so darn easy. Keep in mind, though, that there are three very basic rules that you never, ever want to be guilty of breaking.

Ø TRACKSUIT NO-NO'S:

- ✘ Tight, fitted leggings went out in the eighties and girls, they're not about to a make a comeback.

- ✘ Same goes for stirrups.

- ✘ Panty lines are not cool. Ever. (Need help finding the perfect panties? Read chapter 3, the Panty Shmanty chapter!)

You're all set on tracksuits, then. Don't forget to check out the Shopping Bag chapter in the back of the book to find out where to get the most necessary casual cool wardrobe and more.

CHAPTER 2

workin' it woman

Just because you're busy working at your career doesn't mean your style has to suffer, especially during pregnancy. To keep from falling into that nine-to-five rut, Workin' It Woman shares how to use a few essential pieces to create an amazing work wardrobe. Whether it's a boardroom meeting or casual Friday, *Rock Star Momma* has got you covered. Through the following sections, I'll show you how to get fashionably fabulous work style for all nine months of your pregnancy:

- ★ Straight-Up Suits

- ★ Rockin' Business Casual

- ★ Jet-Set Momma: Biz Travel 101

And remember, while you're busy getting the scoop on how to be a stylish goddess at the office, be sure to check out the **Shopping Bag** chapter in the back of the book to find my most favorite places to go for these must-have nine-to-five looks.

STRAIGHT-UP SUITS

Whether it's every day at the office or that big-shot power lunch, the fact is that most women need to wear a suit or two during their pregnancies. A great suit screams class, elegance, and power. Suits also are—and quite unfortunately—often synonymous with all things stuffy and serious.

Up until now, anyway. I don't want to get weird and political about this, but our mommas went through hell to make motherhood something to be celebrated, not shunned, in the workplace. So let's pay them some respect with outfits that scream sweet, sexy, and strong. Now that *you're* pregnant, it's time to really have fun and show those suits who's boss!

In fact, modern fashion allows for more versatility when it comes to suits. You can now rock your best suit not just at the office, but also at dinner, the theater, at important events— even at weddings. The trick is finding a kick-ass suit that will work from nine to five and then, by simply changing it up with what you wear underneath, shoes, and accessories, it magically becomes appropriate for your after-hours event.

Whatever the occasion, it's pretty safe to assume that a

striking, well-made suit will be a good wardrobe choice. It's a fail-safe option when you just don't know what the heck to wear, since it always looks pulled together and ready for business. Here's how to make them work for you:

★ **Buy Quality:** Don't make the mistake of thinking this only means mucho dinero, but the truth is that when it comes to tailoring, generally speaking, the higher the price tag, the better the fit. And though you're only going to be wearing it for a nine-month stint, you'll wear it a lot, and hey, you've got an impression to make.

★ **Don't Just Think Two-piece:** Most suits are available in the following foundation pieces: jacket, skirt, pants, shift dress, dress coat. Max out the working life of your suit by buying three pieces or more, and then mixing and matching (it'll make getting out of the house every morning soooo much easier, too).

★ **Comfort Is Paramount:** You're going to be wearing that suit for eight, nine, ten-plus hours at a time. Seek out fabrics in breathable-yet-flattering blends of Lycra/spandex, bouclé, cotton/twill, or a light gabardine. You just can't go wrong with any of these, no matter what your office vibe.

★ **Shift into Neutral:** To get the most amount of repeated wear, stick to classic colors like black, navy, camel,

tone it down

Ditch the oversize bag and try a small, understated shoulder bag for those days when you're feeling just too big to deal with the monster bag you're rockin'. Looks great paired with a simple sweater set and classic Mary Janes. Your aching shoulders and back will thank you for the much needed break.

charcoal, or chocolate brown. You can always get bold with shirts, camis, sweaters, shoes, and accessories.

So, now that you have the suit basics down pat, it's time to take a detailed dive into the specifics: Just Jackets, Perfectly Pants, Suitably Skirts, and Ultraglam Underpinnings.

☀ JUST JACKETS

Easily the most important piece of your suited look, since that's what colleagues see when you're at the boardroom table. Worn with matching pants or a contrasting skirt, a suit jacket instantly makes an outfit office-worthy.

Once your pregnant belly pops, the trick to making any suit jacket work is knowing it's okay to let loose and get unbuttoned. Even in the most conservative office, buttons open, please. There are few things worse than a very pregnant lady unpleasantly stuffed into an even stuffier suit. No thank you.

Use this Just Jackets shopping checklist as a helpful guide to finding the best suit jacket for you.

FROM A PRO

Every pregnant gal needs the following essential pieces in her maternity wardrobe:

1. A great white shirt—crisp, clean, and classic—with jeans, a little cleavage, and a great sandal says "sexy weekend," or pair it with an amazing tailored suit and you're still a player in the office.

2. An amazing pair of jeans . . . no explanation needed!

3. Well-fitting black trousers. This can go so many ways . . . it's the "little black dress" of maternity wear.

—KATIE TAGLIAVIA,
owner of 9 Months, key retailer

The Checklist

✓ **Length:** A well-tailored jacket that hits right around the smallest part of your hips will help minimize and flatter in any trimester. If you're on the shorter side, don't go much longer than the top of your thigh, or you'll only look even shorter. Tall gals? With a little bit of height on your side, you've got a few more options. You can easily pull off a longer jacket—one that hits at the thinnest part of your hips, thighs, or even just above your knees. Gotta love the long, lean, and mean jacket for covering up that potentially burgeoning booty, as well. Ah, the secrets of camouflage.

✓ **Cut:** At the start of your pregnancy, you'll look as cool as a cat in a single-breasted jacket with two or three buttons that start just below your bustline. It's the way to go for a sleek, clean look: with a fitted, collared button-up blouse underneath for day or transformed for night over a sexy cami. By the middle to end of your pregnancy, an empire cut is genius for juicing up a classic pair of pants and will beautifully welcome your little intern, too!

✓ **Fit:** The fit of your jacket is crucial to looking clean, neat, stylish, and in control. The perfect fit is one that's slimming, and which accommodates, not accentuates, your expanding frame. As you trot

too hot momma

When shopping for the perfect maternity suit, avoid heavy wool blends, since they'll add unwanted bulk to even the most petite frame, and can be incredibly hot. When those hormones are in overdrive, the result can be an itchy misery. If you do go for wool, make sure it's a light, breathable blend (and check the label for stretch).

FROM DAY TO NIGHT

"A great way to transform an outfit from day to night is with a stylish tube top. Worn under a blazer with a skirt, this outfit is perfect for the office, then take the jacket off to reveal a supersexy outfit for the night out."

—SHANNON DiPADOVA, founder of Due Maternity boutiques and website

through your trimesters, you'll find shoulder seams start to strain. If unbuttoning the jacket doesn't help, consider one that's softly tailored, with a cardigan sleeve. Remember: Long gone are the days of those eighties-inspired, loose, boxy jackets. And no shoulder pads, please . . . you already have enough padding!

☀ PERFECTLY PANTS

These days, pants are the norm in most workplaces. Thank God. Long gone are the days when skirts and pantyhose were a firm requirement (but for those who are still stuck in a skirts-only work world, not to worry . . . just skip ahead to Suitably Skirts). Suit pants offer comfort, conceal those nasty trouble spots, and impart an air of power.

Trouser Power: Here's How to Get It

★   **A Flattering Cut:** You can't go wrong with a straight, boot, or flare leg, no matter how big, small, short, or tall you are. Stick to these basic cuts to get the most wear out of your pants—you'll thank me later.

★   **Go to All Lengths:** A longer cut looks sleek and smart, but a cropped pant cuts to the chase, too, when worn with kitten heels and a crisp button-down. (You can, of course, elevate the look even further with a Birkin bag! Ahhhh . . .) Check out a new favorite in maternity fashion—the gaucho . . . a more fashionable answer to those that are bored with their everyday work trousers.

★ **Fabulous Fabrics:** Some designers call it sharkskin; you know it as superstretchy cotton with a slight sheen. Either way, pants in this fabric are fabulously durable for office wear and tear. Other favorite fabrics to be on the lookout for while shopping: soft, stretch, fine-ply wool and cotton gabardine.

★ **Palazzo No-no:** Terrific for breezing around town on sunny days, a tragedy for looking office-smart. They're floppy and sloppy and they simply just don't work for work.

★ **Waistband Wonders:** Really think about what'll be most comfortable on your waist after an eight-hour workday. The under-the-belly waist is what's going to bring you not only the most comfort, but the most options and longest amount of wear. You'll find good maternity stores/websites stock pants without the dreaded front or side panels, but which contain enough stretch in the fabrics to grow with you.

belly burst

Extend the wear of your regular pants with this handy elastic trick: When trousers start to get too tight, loop a long rubber band around the button, pull it through the buttonhole and back over the button. Works best on side-fastening pants, but a long tank can be your ally on front fasteners. Make sure to conceal this little trick with a longer-fitting blouse!

You just have to check out b-buckles—a stylish, simple elastic band (some are printed with the most clever notions: PEACE, MAMASITA, BUN IN THE OVEN, ROCKSTAR, LOVE, and more) that hooks on the belt loops on both sides of the button and zipper of your pants, allowing you to wear your favorite nonmaternity jeans for just a few more months!

commonsense tip

When it comes to suit pants, ALWAYS remember this— forgo side pockets. They are RARELY flattering, even for you skinny gals! Whatever your shape, side pockets are not the way to go. They just add extra bulk right where you don't want it—in your hips. I also recommend steering clear of most front pleats and tapered legs, both of which only highlight that pear-shape figure you might be sporting just about now.

❊ SUITABLY SKIRTS

The right suit skirt has sex appeal and femininity, while conveying a sense of power and respect. The best length? Right there on the slimmest part of your leg, just below the knee bone—what's known as the "skirt safety zone." When you wear a skirt whose length hits this spot, it's classic, conservative, and, most important, flattering—a win-win every time.

Refer to the **Casual Cool** chapter for the section titled Stellar Skirts. While much of the advice there works for work attire, here's a handful of points to ensure you're office-perfect.

Skirts That Work Checklist

✓ **The Black Staple:** It's slim, it's black, it's flattering, it's versatile. You're not going to make it through your gotta-look-smart-while-pregnant life without it. Trust me.

✓ **Awesome A-line:** It looks great on everyone. Streamline the look with a cashmere twinset. (Keep camis for a slimmer skirt silhouette.)

✓ **Pencil Pro:** Glamorous, slenderizing, and streamlined. Play it up with a don't-mess-with-me turtleneck or matching jacket; soften it with a cable knit or simple shell.

✓ **Clever Linings:** Max out on comfort with soft linings. They'll help your skirt lie flat, conceal any extra baggage that you might be carrying on your backside, and should help hide most panty lines.

Try support hose to conceal cellulite or that unsightly flab you might have going on just about now. Check out the Hot Hosiery section in the **Panty Shmanty** chapter.

A last thought on suit skirts: For the most flattering look, adhere to a balance of power. If you don a skirt that is short and fitted, balance it out with a longer, well-tailored jacket. If it's full and flared, choose a shorter jacket that provides a slim fit. That way, you'll be equally proportioned each and every time.

☀ ULTRAGLAM UNDERPINNINGS

You can change the entire look and feel of your suit just by switching up those underpinnings. Be classically conservative with a collared shirt, downtown diva with a snazzy tank, or straight-up rock star roller with your favorite old concert tee. Here's how you can do it:

★   **Collared Shirt:** A crisp, collared shirt can be cool when you wear it right. Plus, when you're as big as a house, it sure does give you some room to breathe. Use the collar to make a statement—wear it outside of your jacket for a modern nod to John Travolta in *Sat-*

queen of the corporate jungle

Working nine to five doesn't mean you can't experiment with bold prints and textures. Dress up your Monday-through-Friday basics with animal prints and textured fabrics. Both are sexy yet serious enough for the office. And your neutral suits don't have to be tamed! Pair this look with a very modern Lucite or enamel cuff . . . an ultrahip way to loosen up a corporate look!

urday Night Fever. Just like classic JT, it's funky, fun, and always en vogue. Toss on a thick, chunky necklace, strands of pearls mixed with different lengths of silver necklaces, some bold earrings, or sexy shoes to sass it up even more.

★   **T-shirt:** Never thought about a tee under a suit? Think again. Nothing is cooler. A vintage tee, especially one with a little color under a black suit, is chic, playful, and just perfect for an office diva. A classic white fitted tee is timeless, yet understated—ideal for those "I want to be taken more seriously, please" days when paired with a crisp charcoal suit.

Just be sure your tees are flattering and fitted—there's nothing worse than a suit with a too-loose, too-long maternity tee. If you're just starting to pop and that tee is still a little loose, you can clip it or pin it in the back to create a more fitted, more flattering look; the jacket will hide the clip. For more on the best tees for any stage of your pregnancy, go back to the Casual Cool chapter and refresh your memory.

★   **Camisole:** One thing to say about the cami: You can't go wrong. Skin is in, especially when you're pregnant. So show it off! Just use a little discretion when it comes to super-lacy camisoles—some things are best left in the bedroom. If you question its out-of-the-bedroom passability, that cami is probably illegal and best saved for nighty-night time with your man. And don't forget, thinner fabrics show more bulges.

★ **Tank Top:** You gotta love a hot tank top under any suit. Whether it's white, fitted and ribbed, embellished with some vibrant sequins, stones, or other dazzling enhancements, or a punchy bright color such as lime, turquoise, or raspberry, tank tops are sure to add some extra zing to your favorite suit.

Want more accessory advice? You got it. These little add-ons will give any work suit extra sass:

Brooches and pins—a singular sensation that holds a cardigan together in place of boring buttons; a cluster of brooches adds buzz to a lackluster jacket lapel.

Scarves—bonus points for chic when knotted around your neck, threaded through trouser belt loops (only on a low-cut, under-the-belly fit), or twisted around a tote bag handle (SO Gucci!).

Earrings—simple gold or silver hoops, diamond studs, or a cluster of pearls give just the right amount of attitude, while keeping attention where it belongs: not on your earlobes, but on your style.

Watches—an oversize Rolex or men's-style watch, a classic black leather Cartier style, or a striking silver face on a punchy,

accessory tip

It's just amazing how switching up your shoes and handbag can entirely change the look of your suit. A Kelly-inspired bag and professional pumps (I can't believe I just said "pumps"!) create a classy, work-friendly look, while a bohemian clutch and kitten heels create a more playful look that translates from nine-to-five to nighttime in a flash.

pink strap, a watch is more work appropriate than an armload of clunky bracelets.

Necklaces—with a sweater or shirt, an eye-catching, modern-day cameo, string of pearls (I'm really in love with the black variety), or a strand of gold or wood beads. Three necklaces max, at any given time . . . remember, you're at work, girl!

the last word

Finding the perfect pregnancy suit should be a breeze now that you know what to look for—and what to steer clear of. While supertrendy suits in interesting fabrics, embellished sleeves, unique colors, and creative cuts all look really cool when you try them on, forgo the urge and stick with the classics. (Huh? This coming from your trend-obsessed, fashion-worshiping author? Yup, I said it.) Why? Chances are, you're going to wear this suit over and over again for months on end and my bet is that you'll quickly tire of those trendy details—which, by the end of month seven, may no longer be so hip after all. Instead, use accessories and those underpinnings to make your suit into a trendsetting fashion statement that fits your personality and mood. It'll save you time and money in the end.

ROCKIN' BUSINESS CASUAL

Business casual is really a mixed blessing. The plus? It enables you to put a lot of personality, creativity, and thought into your work wardrobe, while affording a lot more comfort and options than traditional suits. The negative? You've actually got to use that creativity and thought to put together those professionally polished yet casual looks.

When you're pregnant, crafting a business-casual wardrobe isn't just about being creative and thoughtful, it's also about having fun and is really quite easy. Honest. You just need to manipulate a few basic pieces to create a lot of looks that are work-worthy each and every time. At the risk of sounding like a Chinese takeout menu, it's all about mixing and matching. I know, I know . . . a lot of fashion-savvy gals have a hard time with that. They want to go to the mall, find an "outfit," and head home. And from that day forward, those pants will forever be married to that shirt to create a single outfit.

Sorry, but when you're a rock star momma, that's just not the way it's done. A rock star momma takes a step back and looks at each piece in her wardrobe as its own little being. When you do that, suddenly that creative switch is turned on and what used to be those three very married, mall-bought outfits easily become nine . . . ten . . . eleven possible outfits— the sky's the limit.

☀ MIX-N-MATCH

Start with a few basics—a pair of suit pants, a matching jacket, a collared shirt, a cami, a cardigan, a skirt, and a great fitted tee—then just mix it up. Pair your suit jacket with a collared shirt and khakis, a couple of necklaces, and some sexy boots on Monday. Team a tee with your suit pants, tie a boldly colored scarf around your wrist, pull your hair back in a ponytail, and don some funky heels for a terrific Tuesday. Toss on a cami, cardigan, and skirt while finishing the look with those sexy knee-high boots for a professional-yet-pretty look on Wednesday. You get the picture.

the last word

⭐ Business casual need not intimidate. Remember, looking great during your pregnancy is all about the right attitude, and when you've got two parts attitude mixed with equal parts confidence, you can pull anything off. Trust in your ability to create—you've already done it once: Just look at that beautiful belly!

JET-SET MOMMA: BIZ TRAVEL 101

Duty calls. Off to New York you go for a major meeting with your biggest account. Only trouble is you're not sure you can fit into the airplane seat—because you're feeling *that* pregnant. Never mind your increasing uncertainty about being able to even pull that carry-on luggage behind you; you're starting to wonder if you and the luggage will both fit down the aisle. Stop worrying, rock star momma. You and your luggage will fit just fine—as long as you pack right.

Think of packing for your business trip as a little experiment. If you can pull this off, getting that bag ready for the hospital will be a breeze (don't worry, though, there's a whole chapter dedicated to just that a little later on). The key is to think simple and remain calm.

✳ ROLLER CHIC

Got a three-day biz trip? All you need is:

★ **A Suit:** It doesn't matter whether it's a pant or skirt suit, but preferably in a stretch cotton so you can scoot off, wrinkle-free, to that meeting the second you touch down.

★ **A Crisp Button-down Shirt:** This works wonders under a suit, with a pencil skirt, and, after hours, with

Take some time to pack your suit-case—don't just shove it all in and pray to the zipper gods that it'll shut. To prevent wrinkling, wrap your clothes in tissue paper. For panties, socks, hosiery, bras, and nightshirts, roll them up. You can stick them in the corners and in random spaces, taking up less room than if you folded them and laid them on top.

supercute jeans and stilettos (always good to pack just in case).

★   A Twinset: Looks business cool for your client lunch and separates out into two versatile pieces for drinks later or just traveling home.

★   A Cami: Under a jacket, with the twinset cardigan or on its own . . . it doesn't even matter if it wrinkles, it just works.

Voilà! Toss them into your roller carry-on and you're done. See ya when you get back.

See how easy it is? You've got that mix-n-match thing mastered now! Going for a few more days? Add a few more pieces, preferably in dark colors so they withstand travel wear-n-tear—and, ick, spills. Going for less? Get rid of something. And there you have it!

❋ ACCESSORIZE, ACCESSORIZE

Plan ahead and think about what kind of accessories speak best to your personal style and the type of biz you're in. Then, pack your faves and bring them along—providing they're light-weight and easy to pack. You'll add some serious panache to your trusty travel garments.

Okay, so that takes care of the suitcase. Now, time to focus on getting YOU ready to head onto the plane. Here are a few tips.

★ **Dress Comfortably:** Say it again: *Dress comfortably*. No need to get fancy anymore, girls—thankfully, dressing up for travel went out a few years back and it's safe to say it's not coming back anytime soon. Rather, think "totally tracksuits," unless you have a meeting to jet off to as soon as you land. If that's the case, then dress as you would for the meeting, choosing a low-wrinkle fabric—matte jersey is perfect since it stretches and holds its shape.

★ **Layer:** A cozy cardigan wrap over a couple of tissue tees makes the perfect travel companion. It'll keep you warm when the temperatures dip, but you can slip it off easily if the mercury soars. And when you've touched down, transition easily from hippie to sleek and subtle sexy with a lightweight, barely buttoned cardigan.

★ **Comfy Shoes:** Whatever your look, wear your very most *comfy shoes*, ones that'll contend with a bit of swelling, because that's more than likely to happen. Pregnancy = swollen feet. Pregnancy + flying = *really* swollen feet. You can always change into your perfect heels when you get into the cab and your feet have had some time to deflate. Thank the shoe gods that the

well-being tip

Now is the time to splurge and book that car service for an easy, hassle-free pickup upon arriving at your destination airport. It will save the aggravation of having to wait in that dreaded cab line, especially after all that travel. Trust me, the extra dough you might spend will be more than worth it! After all, YOU and your little one are worth it and hey, your company might split the bill with you anyway!

i'm with the band

You can do it. Headbands are back and are better than ever! Be sure to wear it about an inch or so off your hairline and allow loose hairs to naturally fall forward. Headbands are great for maintaining a look that's polished, pretty, and sophisticated.

ballet flat has been reincarnated. Ultrafeminine and always stylish, ballet flats are a perfect choice for women on the go. And at last, a chic reprieve from those stilettos you love to hate! Flirty, fun, and easy on your feet, this trend shows no sign of slowing down, so stock up! Trust me, your feet will thank you.

the last word

You're almost set to head off into the sunset . . . or, well, that business trip, anyway. One last little tidbit: Pack a carry-on tote with these key must-have essentials. No matter how long—or short—your flight is, don't leave home without:

- ✓ Your OB/GYN's phone number, just in case.

- ✓ Your ID and travel docs—a no-brainer, I know . . . but then again, you are pregnant and could very well be suffering from pregnesia.

- ✓ A healthy snack, since so few airlines feed you these days and you're eating for two. Try raw nuts and dried fruit . . . yummy!

- ✓ Water, since the low humidity in the cabin causes dehydration. Try to drink at least two liters every two hours to stay hydrated. Very important!

- ✓ A water spray, to spritz over your face and keep you glowing.

✓ Any biz documents—wouldn't want to leave those behind, now, would you?

✓ Breath mints or gum, so that sleepy breath doesn't offend.

✓ Brush and ponytail holder, just in case the seat back ruins your do.

✓ Moisturizer, since the plane ride dries out your skin. It's best to apply a scent-free moisturizer every hour or so to quench thirsty skin. Scent-free, because contrary to popular belief, not everyone wants to be made to smell your new pear-scented lotion.

✓ Shout Wipes, because spills happen, even before Junior arrives.

✓ Travel Blanket—definitely a luxury and not a necessity, I always travel (pregnant or not) with my own blanket so I don't have to use those provided by the airlines. Call me a germ freak, but it's just so much better to bring your own, and it feels great to wrap your precious cargo in a nice, clean—cashmere! if you can—blanket.

✓ Visine—just because you are tired doesn't mean you have to look it.

beauty bag

Let's not forget about your beauty bag essentials! Toss these must-haves into a small case and you're ready as soon as you land: concealer, roll-on perfume, all-in-one blush/bronzer stick, and a juicy tube of lip gloss—the essentials for the two-minute pick-me-up.

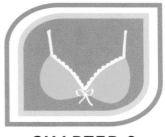

panty *shmanty*

Who doesn't love the way our lingerie makes us feel—whether it's a sexy lace camisole, a great seamless bra, the perfect panty, or those irresistibly quirky low-rider boy shorts that are just right for your favorite jeans.

Up until now, shopping for intimate apparel has been a fun and sexy pastime. But given that you'll probably add between one and two pounds to each breast (the equivalent of squeezing three apples into each cup of your bra!), and your hips, butt, and thighs will swell to unimaginable proportions (so you'll be lucky to even get your favorite G-string over your knees!), it's an absolute necessity.

Surprised? Don't be. The Planet of Mundies (or maternity

undies, by which I mean bras, panties, hosiery), with all its scaffolding and secret compartments, is like a secret world that you're left to navigate all by yourself. It's such a personal place, even closest gal pals don't share their experiences. And sure, it can get a little bit ugly, as well as a little bit hilarious. But, hey, it's gonna be a whole lot more comfortable than what you're wearing right now. So, big breaths (yes, breaths, not breasts! See, you're already in the zone . . .) as you journey through the following sections:

★   Bras, Baby, Bras!

★   Panty Princess

★   Hot Hosiery

FROM A PRO

"After working with thousands of pregnant women, I will tell you that the first thing we always hear is 'Look at this!' (indicating their hips) . . . and then in the next breath . . . turning, 'Look at my butt!' Everyone sees themselves instantly 'flatter,' but we always remind women that it's really just a change in body shape. The best way to battle this early on is with proper underwear! Believe it or not, your old panties now cut into your new hips, generally creating an unsightly panty line . . . gasp . . . and the appearance of butt fat! Combine this with today's slim-fitting, almost always 'no back pocket' maternity pants . . . and panties become a key purchase! And don't forget the bra, ladies! Back fat is just as unsightly! So as your cleavage grows and your ribs spread, check in on a new bra! And the best part is . . . this becomes the perfect reason to splurge at La Perla."

—KATIE TAGLIAVIA,
owner of 9 Months, key retailer

Then check out the Shopping Bag chapter in the back of the book for a must-have list of all the best undie brands and the finest places to shop.

BRAS, BABY, BRAS!

Fact: During your first trimester, a cocktail of hormones conspires to create a network of vessels called milk ducts. As this network grows, so do your breasts. But what also happens is that your breasts become really, REALLY sore; so sore and inflamed that if you even think about putting on a bra, you wince with pain. As for being touched, *fuhgedaboudit*! (This sucks for your partner, because he's so thrilled with your new curves, he can't seem to keep his hands off them. Just tell him to hang in there—it gets better in the second trimester!)

Fact: During your second trimester, those boobs keep on growing, but for most mommas, they're no longer sore or inflamed. This is good news for you, because not only can you go about your everyday life without screaming in agony, but your breasts may even start to feel more sensuous to the touch, which is a bonus for you and your hot-to-trot sweetie.

Fact: During your third trimester, your nipples grow bigger, darker, and firmer, and the blue veins that used to politely live an invisible life beneath the skin may suddenly burst out with a plea to be seen. You see, your breasts are preparing for some serious milk production. In fact, you may even notice your nipples leaking a clear liquid (particularly during foreplay or sex). Nothing to worry about, it's just what's known as colostrum, a type of premilk.

Fact: During the postpartum "fourth trimester," your breasts do things they never did before: they make milk. And for the first week or so after delivery (whether you decide to breast-feed or not), they will become rock-hard and heavy and, once again, very uncomfortable.

Needless to say, during each of the trimesters of pregnancy, your breasts are changing. Even gals who've been flat as pancakes can grow at least two bra sizes during their pregnancy. So with this radical transformation in mind, it just makes sense that you'll need a few new bras.

I highly recommend you invest in a great maternity bra. Yes, it'll be more $$$ than a bigger, regular bra, but these bras are designed for every aspect of your blossoming bod—from your expanding rib cage to the increasing strain on your chest muscles. And make sure to get measured by a professional. In the long run, she'll save you money.

FOR ALL YOU SEXY MOMMAS

Supermodel Elle Macpherson designed her own maternity bra for Elle Macpherson Intimates (an incredibly gorgeous lingerie collection) when, as a nursing mom, she couldn't find a bra that was pretty, feminine, and practical. The collection includes two *fabulous* maternity bras: La Mere and the Maternelle. Both bras are lined with 100 percent cotton for maximum comfort. And you definitely won't compromise any style or sex appeal with these beauties!

The La Mere style is *stunning* and is the ultimate bra for new moms. You'll love the stretchy-yet-sturdy fabrics and construction of both styles. There's more of Elle in our Postpartum Panache chapter, where you'll learn everything you need to know about nursing bras!

Now, use this Pregnancy Bra Shopping Checklist to ensure you've hit the right fit.

The Checklist

✓ **Check the Straps:** They should be wide-set, thick in width, and lie flat against your back. If the straps dig into your skin or your skin hangs over the band, your bra is already too small. Although to contradict myself here, the newest crop of pregnancy bras are surprisingly dainty and not terribly wide in the strap region.

✓ **Support:** Now is just not the time to go braless. In fact, good support now minimizes stretch marks later, since skin layers are less likely to pull and separate. Plus, it helps prevent saggy banana breasts later. Oh, momma! Look for a wide underband, which will provide the scaffolding you need as your breasts get heavier and is a hundred times more comfortable than underwire (ouch!). What else? Read on . . .

✓ **Cups:** The softer, the better. The cup shouldn't wrinkle or pucker; it should lay smooth, so avoid seamed cups, too. You might be tempted to go for a prettier, sexier half cup. Don't. A full cup will give more support, ease discomfort, and help avoid not-so-sexy stretch marks down the road.

✓ **Fabric:** A blend of 92 percent cotton/8 percent spandex is perfect for allowing the cups to mold to your breasts and offers all-day comfort and support. Because cotton lets your skin breathe, it's the best fabric for your breasts! (Bras with 100 percent cotton lining are definitely a plus!) And, who can be bothered with hand washing? Cotton is sturdy enough to throw into the machine every couple of days. (But I say hang-dry those bras if you want them to truly hold their shape!)

✓ **Hooks:** Adjustable hooks are key—as your back widens, you'll need to use those different hooks for comfort. Look for at least three hooks, even four. Buy the bra that fits comfortably when fastened using the hooks farthest in.

✓ **Sleep:** During your third trimester—when your breasts are nearing their biggest—it's a great idea to sleep in a jog bra to provide 24/7 support. Now is the time to use maximum support to help combat drooping later!

✓ **Colors:** The best bra color is the one that matches your skin: stock up on them. They'll go with everything—from the sheerest white T-shirt (never wear a white bra with a white T-shirt—it'll show right through) to the sexiest of camisoles. Stock up on a couple great daytime maternity bras to get you through your pregnancy, while investing in one or two "special occasion" bras for those special nights. Black or lace, anyone?

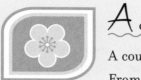 ## A Little Secret

A couple of random thoughts from me here. From the moment I found out I was pregnant, I wore a bra all day, every day . . . 24/7! I just felt better—not only from being a heck of a lot more comfortable, but somewhere deep in my head, I had convinced myself that if I did so, I would avoid stretch marks around my boobs. I bought a couple different types of bras—from the straight-up sports bra to those sheer tank-style bras (sans the underwire) to the half-lace, half-shiny silky bra top. I stopped wearing all my old bras, which were near to no longer fitting, and horribly uncomfortable with the stiff underwire, and went with one of my new-school bras that I fell in love with instantly. And let me tell you this—I have NO stretch marks there, or anywhere else for that matter!

HELP???

 "How can I purchase a nursing top or bra now when I know my body might change after I have my baby? is a question I get often. I answer by telling them that most women increase two cup sizes after delivery and that they should purchase a bra that will work for them before and after baby arrives."*

—GERMAINE CAPRIO,
founder of Majamas

fashion tip

Make your favorite nonmaternity bras last longer by using a bra back extender. This handy little contraption is an extender that you clasp onto the hooks of your bra to increase its band width, anywhere from an inch to over three inches. This is great if your bras still fit in the cup, but are getting tight around your back and under your bust. Bra back extenders help you get by with your old bras for at least a few weeks, if not longer. You can find them in most department stores and maternity boutiques. Check out the **Shopping Bag** chapter in the back of the book for more info!

CELEB FAVORITE!

By far the most innovative and comfortable bra ever—the iBra by Wacoal, a completely stitchless, seamless, and tagless contour bra. Sleek, sexy, and sophisticated. Can you say "AHHHHHH . . ."? The innovative design of the iBra approaches comfort from the inside out, focusing on every point of contact that a bra makes with the body. By eliminating stitches and seams, the iBra leaves nothing but a smooth fabric surface against the body. The underwire is comfortably hidden and sealed between fabric layers, so there is never any exposed wire or stitching against the body. It's no wonder that so many leading ladies LOVE this thing!

❋ NURSING BRAS 101

Your baby has finally made its way into the world and if you've decided to breast-feed, you've got a whole new bag of issues to deal with: nursing bras. When you're nursing, you want a bra that allows easy access while offering tons of support.

There are three major factors to keep in mind when selecting a nursing bra:

★ **Fabric:** As your breasts fill with milk, they grow and grow and grow. Until it's time for a feeding . . . and then they shrink right back down. To accommodate this constant change in size, it's best to have a nursing bra that's made with at least 5 percent spandex. This provides excellent moldability, so as your breasts change size, it continues to support and ease discomfort, and allows room for milk-absorbing nursing pads.

★ **Fit:** A nursing bra should fit you perfectly, so seek the help of a professional. A bra that's too small can inhibit the flow of milk and result in pain, engorgement (when ducts get blocked), or worse, infection.

★ **Accessibility:** When nursing, you'll want a bra that's all about easy access. Invest in a bra that not only offers easy access for Junior, but that's just as easy for you to manipulate, wherever you may be. Whether it's a sports bra, one with a front clasp, pull-down cups, or easy lifting, the start of month eight is the time to try on numerous bras until you find the one that's most user-friendly for you.

Just like for pregnancy bras, you'll want to purchase three nursing bras for daytime and one for going out at night (yes, you will eventually go out at night again!). Remember, you'll need to stock up on nursing pads to prevent leaks, too. In fact, when you go to try on nursing bras, bring a set of nursing pads with you, to ensure a true fit.

Check out the double-banded elastic-front nursing bra by Japanese Weekend. It's soft, stretchy, and easy to use. There are no hooks, no itchy, scratchy Velcro; it's so comfortable you can sleep in it. Many moms do! This bra works with just about

quick sizing tip
The bra you're wearing in the last two months of pregnancy should be your starting point. Choose a nursing bra with the same band size (that's the number, ladies!), but bump up one cup size—yes, that's the letter! So for example, if you are a C in your final months of pregnancy, best bet is to get a D nursing bra.

any body type, so feel confident that you're going to love this bra. Don't forget to check out the **Postpartum Panache** chapter for everything you need to know about nursing bras.

PANTY PRINCESS

Ah, the choices! G-string, bikini, French brief, tap pant, boy short, low rider, hip hugger, Brazilian, seamless, over the belly. Thankfully, panties have come a long way for maternity mavens. These days it's all about personal preference. Like 'em lean and low? Hip-hugging thongs for you, my dear. Like 'em sexy, but with full coverage? Lace boy shorts should do the trick. Classic simplicity? Straight-up cotton bikinis are calling your name.

Panty Princess is all about "sexy practicality." It's important that you feel like the sexy goddess you are while keeping comfort a priority, as well. To help you do so, check out this handy guide to help you choose perfect panties. It might not be Agent Provocateur, but it's sure worth trying!

THE ROCK STAR momma'S GUIDE TO THE PERFECT PREGNANCY PANTIES

Comfort: There is just nothing worse than uncomfortable panties, especially when you're pregnant, when even the littlest things can drive you crazy. So why do the battle? Ask not-so-prissy girlfriends what worked for them, but we say, buy what's comfiest for you . . . even if you end up with a drawer full of granny pants!

The Land Down Under: As you make way for baby, you're going to put on some weight. For some gals, it's the required twenty-five to thirty-five pounds and for others it's upward of fifty, sixty, even seventy pounds. You're also bound to retain water. That means your once well-fitting panties are likely to become too tight. Read on for tips on what to look for to achieve a perfect panty fit:

- ✓ *No-riders:* When your panties ride up, that's a serious no-no and means that they're too small. Bump up a size (again, no pun intended).

- ✓ *Under-the-belly:* Make sure that if you're carrying your baby really low, your panties ride low. Hip huggers and low-rise thongs are good choices for you.

- ✓ *The digs:* Be sure that your panties don't do "the digs," that is, when they dig into your sides and leave red marks behind on your hips. This happens mostly with G-strings and string-bikini bottoms. To prevent the digs, invest in panties that will give you some breathing room. Lots of stretch!

Fabric: When it comes to fabric, knock yourself out and get as crazy as Victoria's Secret, Cosabella, or Agent Provocateur will let you. Cotton is the way to go—it's always the most comfortable! But whatever fabrics you choose, be sure that they really feel good on your skin. Also, as a rule of thumb, the "gusset"—a fancy word for "crotch"—should always be 100 percent cotton to allow for breathability, absorption (you don't want to hear it, but your vaginal discharge is going to increase), and to help avoid irritation.

No More Panty Lines: Gals, there is nothing worse than panty lines! Do not fall victim to this easily preventable fashion faux pas. They are just NOT okay, and should never have to happen! When in doubt, always, always turn to seamless bikini or thong panties in a nude color that matches your skin tone. Now, if only those "don'ts" in the back of *Glamour* magazine were reading this right now . . .

Alrighty, now that you know how to find the perfect pair of pregnancy panties, how the heck are you supposed to know which ones to wear with what? It's quite simple, really! Just use this handy-dandy chart for the maximum in maternity style, comfort, sexiness, and, of course, panty line—free looks.

IF YOU WEAR THESE BOTTOMS:	THEN WEAR THESE PANTIES:
Low-riding maternity jeans	Low-rise boy briefs
Loose, drawstring skirts	G-strings or thongs
Fitted maternity skirts	Seamless briefs or thongs
Dressy maternity pants	Seamless briefs, G-strings, or thongs
Sexy maternity sundresses	Lace-trimmed boy shorts
Short, ruffled minis	Lace-trimmed boy shorts
Maternity suits	Seamless briefs or thongs
Workout apparel	Seamless briefs, bikinis, G-strings, or thongs
Drawstring cargo pants	Seamless briefs, G-strings, or thongs

So, there you have it, panty princess. It doesn't matter whether you get your panty stash at Target or Bergdorf Goodman. What matters is that you find a great fit that can grow with your pregnancy, even on your most bloated, irritable days, in fabrics that feel good against your skin and cover the right things at the right times. Got it? Great! Moving on . . .

⭐ HOT HOSIERY

Ugh. Wearing pantyhose pretty much sucks, but for many, it's still an unfortunate requirement in the everyday workplace. When you're pregnant, hormonal, bloated, puffy, and uncomfortable, the last thing you want to do is stuff yourself into a pair of pantyhose. While you may be craving sausage, you certainly don't want to feel like one.

Fortunately, pantyhose companies are making huge strides in the comfort arena, specifically for pregnant women. The newest thing? Compression hosiery. Compression hosiery is designed to massage and support your legs in the areas where you need it so that circulation is increased and swelling is reduced. As always, check with your doctor first, as compression hose might not be recommended for you. You can wear them over or under the belly, and the result is a slimmer appearance that makes you feel less claustrophobic and more comfortable. I gotta tell you, you won't win a beauty pageant with these things, but are you really trying? If you have achy leg issues and feel the need for more support, I say go online and Google away!

Thigh-highs are also a great alternative to traditional hose when you're pregnant. They're sexy, sultry, and, thankfully, they come nowhere near your belly. Get the right fit, though, because you don't want your thigh-highs too tight or too loose. You don't want to cut off your circulation, but you also don't want your hosiery falling down your legs by lunch hour.

When choosing hosiery for your pregnancy, choose a hue that's sheer for professional occasions. Get the tone that's closest to your skin color—the idea is to match your skin tone, not to make you look tan or ghostly.

For fun, flirty outfits—like a ruffled miniskirt paired with a fitted, shape-hugging turtleneck—black tights are best. Paired with a great pair of boots or some sexy heels, you'll instantly add class and sass while appearing slimmer.

FROM A PRO

"Doctors actually recommend wearing comfy support hosiery during pregnancy because they improve circulation, prevent varicose veins, and provide back and underbelly support. And for many celebrity moms-to-be who have to jet around the world promoting their favorite flick, many doctors recommend wearing supportive hosiery on airplanes."

—SARA BLAKELY,
founder of Spanx

fake-n-bake

Skip the pantyhose and instead apply some self-tanner to get that smooth, bronzed look that we all know and love. Plus, while you may be feeling rather pallid, having a faux glow is the perfect way to make you look like a million bucks—even when you're not feeling like it. Just follow these easy steps to get the perfect tan:

- Exfoliate in the shower with a moisturizing scrub.
- To help ensure a smoother application, apply a layer of moisturizer first.
- Apply self-tanner in a circular motion, starting at the top of your feet and working your way up.
- Avoid elbows, knees, and heels for a streak-free tan.

Try these: Babor self-tanning lotion, Mystic Tan aerosol tan spray, and California Tan self-tanning lotion. And as always, talk to your doc before using any of these products!

Fishnets are a fabulously sexy option for pregnancy hosiery, too. Pair with a simple sheath, an A-line skirt, or go for the knee-high kind under jeans with some sexy heels. Foxy lady!

☀ HOSIERY KNOW-HOW

Thanks to Sara Blakely and Spanx, the amazing hosiery line with specialty maternity stockings, comfort, support, and quality have arrived! Mama Spanx full-length and footless pantyhose deliver a cradle of comfort for expectant mommas. Spanx features a nonbinding (read: comfortable and wearable) waistband and added underbelly support. And be sure to check out their new pregnancy-friendly bra with absolutely *no* metal . . . can you say "thank GOD!"?

Ø HOSIERY NO-NO'S

✘ **Printed or Patterned Hosiery:** When you're pregnant, you've got MORE than enough going on. This is the one time when you don't want to use bright, bold-patterned prints to make a statement.

✘ **Too-tan Hosiery:** Don't even try to fake a tan by engaging in too-tan hosiery. Stick to self-tanners (see sidebar).

✘ **White Tights:** They weren't a good look before you were pregnant. Now that your legs are looking a little bloated, what makes you think they're a good look now? You don't? Whew, just checking . . .

✗   **Stockings and Garter Belts:** This sizzling combo may have sent his temperature soaring before week twelve. By your second trimester, you'll just look like a badly strung guitar! Hi-larious. Plus, who needs all that extra technology around the tummy? Don't go there— even if your rock star papa likes badly strung guitars.

the last word

Panty shmanty! You've made your way through the world of maternity bras, underwear, and more, and hopefully you now have the knowledge to create a beautiful, functional, comfortable, and sexy maternity lingerie collection. The most important things to remember? Fit, feel, and form. But no matter what you wear, always remember that you are a sexy, strong rock star momma!

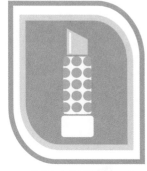

head-to-toe *glow*

First the good news: There will be days during your pregnancy when you are the embodiment of what's known as "the bloom." In other words, your hair will be shinier than the sun, your skin will be clear and glowing, your teeth will sparkle, your eyes will twinkle, and you'll generally look so radiant, so blooming, passersby will probably rush up to you and shower you with compliments . . . before asking for your autograph.

Now the bad news: There will also be days when you feel as blooming as a dandelion caught in the firing line of a passing cat. That you may have spent the morning, poor thing, throwing up is only the start of it. No matter what you do, your hair will appear to have a mind of its own, your skin has erupted into a barrage of blemishes, and, *quelle horreur,* is that the shadow of a mustache you're starting to see? And, despite an extra precautionary layer of antiperspirant, your armpits are producing more H_2O than a power shower . . .

Listen, even Kate and Debra had their good and bad days. (Luckily for most of us, we don't have the paparazzi recording those moments of our pregnancy we'd rather forget.) No one (and that includes Britney and any other woman with more money than Uggs) is immune to the effects of hormones gone haywire on our hair, skin, teeth, nails . . . even body aroma. And everyone is entitled to feel conflicted at times about their expanding belly, as well as breasts, thighs, ankles . . . and even neck (don't ask).

But here's the lesson to be learned: When you focus on embracing your new, ever-changing bod and the baby you're creating, not even scaly skin or overactive armpits can ruin your mood for long. Relish and revel in the days when you look and feel like a rockin' hot momma-to-be. And on the days you don't, well . . . use even the smallest annoyance as a big excuse for pampering and splurging on a treat you know will improve the way you look and feel about yourself.

Coming up, you'll learn of the biggest beauty blahs you're likely to meet en route to rock star mommahood—and the simple strategies that'll keep you glowing. Check them out:

★   Tress Distress

★   Complexion Perfection!

★ Your Hot Bod

★ Pamper Yourself

Star Style: Mariska Hargitay

"There are no beauty tricks! Being pregnant gives you a glow that can't be found in a bottle. But really, everyone is so busy staring at your belly, you're lucky if they even look at your face. Embrace it all. The swollen feet, the rosy cheeks, the waddling, the endless bloody noses, the nausea, the constant hunger, and I mean constant, the moments at four a.m. when you would pay any amount of money just to find a comfortable position and go to sleep, the weird cravings, the complete failure of your abs. . . . But living for nine months with two heartbeats (or more!) makes all of it so unbelievably worth it."

TRESS DISTRESS

If you were obsessed with your hair before you became pregnant (who isn't?), you'll be certifiable now that you're with babe. Because the hair you thought you knew is, by your fourth month, a complete stranger. Thanks to all those crazy-fabulous reproductive hormones increasing your blood circulation and metabolism, your hair may be growing faster than wildfire. If it used to be fine and flyaway, it might now look thicker, too—it's down to those hormones again, stopping the natural shedding process.

Many women encounter a major attack of the greasies early on, then spend their second and third trimesters fighting the dry and frizzies! Once thick, luscious locks may start to look wispier, and stick-straight hair can suddenly turn curly— and vice versa. Either way, hang on to your helmet . . . during pregnancy, you and your hair are going to experience some turbulence.

HAIR HELP

First Trimester Hair Horror

Your follicles are freaking out, thanks to the flood of estrogen that's made its way to your hair. If you're lucky, almost overnight you'll have a mane to die for (y'know . . . thick, shiny, and loads of volume). If you're unlucky, you'll wake up one day to an out-of-control, flyaway, foresty mess. Reduce the mayhem with this *Rock Star Momma* Hair RX:

★ *Shampoo Swap*

See all those products lined up along your bathroom shelf? Good-byeee! Few women really consider the chemical quotient in their shampoos and conditioners before they conceive. Now that you're pregnant— and going through hair hell—it's time to swap highly scented, deluxe foaming hair cleansers for super-gentle products that still get the job done (remember, during those early months, your hair may well be greasier and, therefore, may attract more dirt). You don't need a master's in pharmaceuticals, just look for products suitable for "fragile" or "stressed" hair or "color-treated hair."

★ *Condition It*

Whether your hair's suddenly gone greasy or dull and dry, keep conditioner close by. If your pregnancy hair's oily or limper than William Hung's handshake, choose a light, gel-based conditioner. Oily hair still needs moisture and protection from the elements and pollution, but the treatment needs to be light. Creamy conditioners will only drag it down. Save those creamy, opaque concoctions for dry hair—if it's turned frizzy, too, look for conditioning creams that contain collagen or silk. And treat your confused tresses to a weekly conditioning mask—feels so good. (Feels even better when you're simultaneously receiving a foot massage from your beloved.)

Second Trimester Hair Horror

Your roots are seriously starting to show. You have been so diligent about not coloring your hair during the first trimester (that all-important time when your baby's brain is developing), you've avoided any salon within a fifteen-mile radius. Trouble is, you're now starting to look like you're wearing a brown—or some other not-so-hot—skullcap. You thought you could handle reuniting with your natural hair color, but guess what? You CAN'T! Okay, calm down . . . here's your Hair RX:

★ *Know the Facts*

As always, once you're in full possession of the facts, it's easier to make decisions about whether to color your hair during pregnancy—or not. Truth is, dear rock star momma, the facts are a little muddy. One study (in 1998) found that hair dye was associated with about a 3 percent greater chance of delivering a baby with a specific type of heart defect. That said, it didn't conclude that the hair dye caused the defect. In fact, it had the lowest risk increase of all the factors they tested, including pesticides, cleaning solvents, and certain medications. Most of us who color—or, God forbid, perm—our hair will have done so before we even knew we were pregnant. And what experts agree on is this: Even if you did, the very minimal amount of chemicals that are absorbed into the skin during the coloring or perming process is not enough to cause a problem for your developing baby. Still, I say if you can help it, why risk it? So . . .

★ *Find an Alternative Fix*

You could wear a hat for the next six, five, four, or so months. But it's far cooler (by at least five degrees) to consider highlights—or a variation such as lowlights, or even paint-on hair color—since they're usually applied at least a half inch away from your scalp, so there's very little chance the chemicals will enter your bloodstream. You should also ask your stylist about semipermanent or vegetable dyes that are low on chemicals (although, with the exception of henna, not completely chemical-free). You won't achieve exactly the same hair color you've been used to, but they do camouflage outgrowth pretty well, particularly if you use a color-enhancing shampoo, too.

Third Trimester Hair Horror

Static, static . . . and more s-s-s-static. So you've shampooed gently and conditioned like crazy and resisted the urge to chop off all your hair at week thirty-six . . . along comes static just to push you screaming one step closer to hair insanity. *Argh!!* Chances are it'll creep up on you in your third trimester. Why? Your little bundle of fun is having one last growth spurt before bursting through your waters—and consuming as much liquid as possible, depleting your body's supplies of *eau* from every corner, including your hair! The drier your skin and hair becomes, the more prone you are to static electricity. And if it's winter, too? Oh, boy, you'd better love high hair!! So here's your Hair RX:

perm point of view

In short, no, no, no! They're just plain bad for your scalp (that fixation solution can cause irritation and soreness and hasn't been proven to be risk-free for developing babies) and bad for your hair (think damaged and desert dry), and a really bad look, period. So, please, definitely not now. Not ever.

★ *Drink Gallons of Water*

See that large bottle of Evian? Drink it. And then some more.

★ *Let Us Spray*

Buy some leave-in conditioner or hair spray or anti-static spray and blast it on your brush before you style.

★ *Add Vinegar*

Although your heightened sense of smell will most likely loathe the smell of vinegar almost as much as you loathe static (but not quite), add a few drops of vinegar to your final cool-water rinse after washing. Honestly, it'll help.

❋ STYLE IT, SISTAH!

Emotions and mood swings during pregnancy can cause you to make all sorts of rash decisions: from wanting to rearrange every room in your house to trying a completely different hairstyle. And if your once-glorious head of bouncing curls has turned into stick-straight straw, you may even be considering cutting it all off! Wooooooooooah . . .

A radical hair transformation is risky at the best of times, but when your girth is twice its normal size, *fuhgeddaboudit.* Trust me, body versus head proportion has a lot to do with hair style success, and your proportions are changing every week . . . and will certainly change dramatically all over again by week forty (remember?).

Look, if your hair is driving you crazy and you're craving a change, think temporary, think work-with-what-you-have, think BEAUTY NIGHT!

QUICK FIX

★   A little goes a long way: If your hair's normally straight, give it a wave (you gotta try those cute 100 percent cotton, machine-washable hair twists from Mark Garrison that produce gentle waves in under twenty minutes); if it's normally curly, experiment with flat irons. If you normally wear your long hair down, get a girlfriend or your mom to help you pin it up. Small changes can make a big difference.

★   Most stylists will come to your home for the same fee they'd charge at the salon. Book one you already know for a couple of hours for an en masse blowout for you and your best girlfriends. Or . . .

★   Ask your stylist for a subtle change, such as layers, bangs, or texturizing. Remember: Shorter styles only accentuate weight gain. Start with soft layers around your face. If those work, then get a little more adventurous.

Keep It Real

I admit, I sometimes allow my vanity to get in the way, but this time it was all about the baby, and this lady—ME—wasn't going to risk it in ANY WAY. Translated, that meant my "enhanced" blonde locks were slowly (or not so slowly) turning to the dark side. Believe me, I really wanted to color my hair as scheduled, but my better judgment just said to wait. So I did. I didn't touch my hair and I was going nowhere near a salon where I could breathe in anything chemical. (Okay, I admit it now, I was a little neurotic!) Finally, I allowed a colorist friend to color my hair with an all-natural process—in an empty salon—and give me a couple of highlights here and there. And it worked! It wasn't what I normally do, but it gave me a lift—in color and mood—that I needed. But only you will know what you're comfortable doing. Run with your instincts.

Blow, Baby, Blow!

Try a blow-dryer brush like the one from Revlon—the Ionic Hot Air Dryer and Styler (only twenty bucks and can usually be found at a local drugstore—if not, there's always the Internet!). It's small, quick, and easy to use. This dandy little thing uses ion technology—translated: better for your hair and dries faster, with fuller, silkier results. You'll end up with smooth styles, curves, and bouncy waves. AND the ionic charge also helps get rid of static, thus reducing frizz. Try brushing hair upward, pulling straight up above your head as you roll ends under. This will give you added volume at the roots. There's nothing wrong with that!

COMPLEXION PERFECTION!

Along with extra pampering from your sweetie, permission to burst into tears when stuff (*anything!*) doesn't go your way, a whole new reason to go shopping, and a credible excuse to eat plenty of ice cream (calcium is so good for your developing fetus, as well as you), along comes indescribably fabulous skin to add to the bountiful list of benefits of being pregnant. Hooray!

Yup, there will be times when your complexion will literally *glow*! You'll look as though you've spent a fortune on Armani's Luminous Silk Foundation (the best, right?), topped off with Stila's utterly entrancing range of eye-brightening shadows and kissable lip glosses. In fact, the truth is you will probably have just fallen out of bed. Aside from simply being so darn happy about your new baby news, this au naturel glow is thanks to increased blood flow to the vessels just beneath the surface of your skin, and pregnancy hormones that cause your oil glands to release more than usual so your face looks divinely dewy.

But just so you don't get thoughts above your station (i.e., seriously considering becoming a supermodel), the goddess of pregnancy has decreed that there will also be times when you will break out, blotch up, and/or turn unusually brown. For crying out loud, don't panic. It's all perfectly normal momma-to-be skin behavior. And, happily, all temporary and fixable, too. So come away from the mirror, stop squeezing (repeat: stop squeezing), fretting, poking, and sobbing—and read on.

☀ COMPLEXION (IM)PERFECTIONS

From A(cne) to Z(its)

There's no predicting whether you're going to be plagued with pimples or blessed with blemish-free skin during your nine

"Contrary to what loved ones say, many women do not experience that special 'glow' during pregnancy. As hormones change, the skin is naturally affected. In fact, some women experience unbalanced skin ranging from a dull, uneven appearance to full-blown breakouts. While women need an effective skin-balancing cleanser, many contain ingredients like benzoyl peroxide and salicylic acid that should be avoided during pregnancy. Try the BASQ Rebalancing Cleanser, which addresses these problems in an effective way that is safe and gentle enough for use during pregnancy. It contains oak root extract with natural tannins that have mild astringent and antiseptic qualities to soothe irritated, unbalanced skin. Ylang-ylang, an exotic flower blossom, is blended in to smooth the appearance of skin for a revitalized and refreshed 'glow.'"

—KELLI KENNY AND LAUREN PARISIER,
cofounders of Basq

months. Some women suffer all their lives with problem skin, then become pregnant, and presto!, they don't see a single spot for their entire term. Other women, who may have boasted a clear complexion their whole lives, can wake up one day and discover they have more pimples than a pack of Boy Scouts. It's a lottery!

What tends to happen is that rising levels of your hormone-y friends, estrogen and progesterone, stimulate your sebaceous glands and cause them to produce more oil. When the oil becomes trapped in the pores, bacteria starts to feast on it, the area becomes inflamed, and, well, you will end up with either a little zit or full-blown acne, depending on how much oil and how blocked the pore is and how long it's blocked.

You should already know about the many benefits of exfoliation. And face masks. And . . . mmmm . . . facials. Deep cleansing and regular removal of old skin cells, which help declog pores and encourage new skin cells to come to the surface, is your credit card to a clear complexion, pregnant or not. But what many rock star mommas don't know is that regular skin regimes can become risky when you're expecting.

Skin Swap #1

By the time you're ready to have a baby, chances are you've left teen exfoliators behind and progressed onto more hi-tech (and expensive) products that contain a plethora of ingredients with fancy-sounding names such as alpha hydroxy acid, or AHAs. Okay, stop right there! While there's no evidence to suggest AHAs are bad for developing babies, one reason *zit tip*

Try dabbing on toothpaste—yes, toothPASTE, not the gel type, it has to be the pasty type—to help with those unexpected zits. It calms them down and dries them out overnight. Just remember to wash it off before you answer the door or walk the dogs the next morning! (Hot compresses work wonders, too, and are very calming.)

women love their effect on troubled skin is that they have the power to penetrate deep, deep, deep—and that's why some doctors advise limiting use when pregnant. It's especially important to keep exfoliating now, so you have two other options: Look for exfoliators with an AHA content of less than 5 percent (Avon Anew, for example) or try one that's completely AHA-free (suggestions: Ling's Honey & Almond Facial Scrub and Rodan + Fields Reverse exfoliate: micro-dermabrasion paste).

Skin Swap #2

Serious acne can tempt you to take drastic measures, but no doctor in her right mind should prescribe you an oral medication such as Accutane, or retinoic acid, when you're pregnant. In fact, the FDA doesn't recommend trying to get pregnant for one month after you stop taking Accutane. Taking Accutane will clear your acne, but it'll also give your baby a 35 percent greater chance of birth defects, such as mental retardation, brain malformation, heart defects, or facial abnormalities. It also increases your chance of miscarriage. This is serious and just not worth the risk. Treat your acne instead from the outside. But experts even caution against our usual over-the-counter favorites such as all retinol products, salicylic acid, or benzoyl peroxide. Instead, here's a little Hollywood secret: Sonya Dakar's totally natural Drying Potion. It tingles slightly when you first dab it on and, thanks to the zinc oxide, it forms a white crust (sex-ay!), but it contains no risky ingredients whatsoever. Used overnight, this stuff's a true rock star momma complexion lifesaver.

Dry, Dry, Baby

Having said your sebaceous glands will start to pump out more oil than the state of Texas in your first trimester, by your second or third, dry patches become a big issue. Developing babies require lots of fluids and, if necessary, they'll siphon off the moisture in your skin and hair to get it. What's more, just as you've grown nauseated by foods you previously loved, your rock star momma skin may develop sensitivities to your favorite face products.

So what's the good news, you're asking? (I know, all these changes can be overwhelming, but hang on . . .) The good news is . . . um . . . no, seriously, the good news is that there are plenty of divine products that are also natural and gentle. Avoid soap altogether and, instead, try out a milk-based or creamy cleanser that softens as it cleans. *Rock Star Momma* recommendation: one that's fragrance free but has a goopy, custard-thick texture to satisfy your need for pampering. You'll love La Roche-Posay, which is perfume and preservative-free.

Next, replace your usual toner with an alcohol-free, soothing, and hydrating rosewater or witch hazel. Or just skip straight to moisturizing cream (more effective than lotion). When you dab it onto damp skin, it locks even more moisture in.

Talking of drinking . . . guzzling water is actually the best remedy for dry skin. Keep a bottle on your desk, in your tote, by your bed. And when you're not drinking it, spray it on your face—Evian and Almay make the best facial water mists. Try storing in the fridge so they feel fabulously cool and soothing on superhot days. Now, *that's* good news.

The Dreaded Mask

You've probably heard the horror stories already, but there's no getting away from it: chloasma or melasma or the "pregnancy mask" (call it what you want) is pretty common. In fact, up to 70 percent of pregnant women experience it to some degree.

Normally starting in your second trimester, hormone activity makes the pigment-producing skin cells (known as melanocytes) hypersensitive to sunlight. The result? Brown, splotchy patches on the face and body, usually over your chin, cheeks, nose, top lip, and forehead.

Listen, it's all very well for those other pregnancy books to tell you not to get upset about the mask, but the truth is, no, it doesn't look great. Yes, it will disappear after delivery—thank God—but, rock star momma, I know you wanna look your best *now.* Right?

Here's what you can do: Stay out of the sun. Hibernate. Go to bed and don't get up for nine months. Yeah, right. Meanwhile, back in the real world (and yours!) . . . immediately, as soon as you're pregnant if not before, invest in a really good sunscreen. Check out the Anti-Chloasma Facial Sunscreen SPF 25 from Belli. It's rich but not too cloggy for the face, totally allergy tested, and smells absolutely gorgeous!

Also, be religious, *fanatical* about folic acid. Studies have shown those women who consume plenty of vitamin B not only ensure the healthy development of their growing baby, but reduce the risk of the dreaded mask, too. So pile your plate with spinach, broccoli, and whole grains.

If, despite everything, brown patches appear, get clever with foundation and concealer. Your usual shade probably won't give enough coverage, so, hey, what's a girl to do except experiment with a makeover at her nearest MAC counter? Since all the associates are trained makeup artists, they give great advice and I've found they have the best range of creamy concealer shades that don't give that gross "pancake" makeup vibe. Know what I mean? Also, check out MAC's line of makeup made from all mineral-based ingredients.

> ## SUNSCREEN GOSPEL
>
>
>
> "It's important to look for either avobenzone or zinc oxide as the main active ingredients in a sunscreen, because these ingredients block out UV light, the wavelength that causes these big ugly brown patches."
>
> —KATIE RODAN, M.D.,
> dermatologist and cofounder of
> Rodan + Fields

☀ PICTURE PERFECT

Want flawless skin?…You got it, and it's easier than you think. Follow these easy steps and you're on your way to a simply stunning look: *Keep in mind, I always recommend mineral makeup as there's no doubt that it's better for your skin right now.*

* ★ **Concealer:** Just what you'll need to cover the dark spots from the dreaded "pregnancy mask." Also, great

beauty buy tip

Try the Vincent Longo cream con- cealers—experi- ment with blending shades for a perfect skin tone match. This stuff lasts all day and is so light, yet extremely effec- tive at covering everything from dreadful pregnancy mask to an- noying zits to spider veins!

for covering up the dark circles you might have from restless nights. Yellow tones are perfect for this. And make sure that your concealer is always slightly lighter than your foundation. I love the stick kinds that are super easy to apply and mess-free.

★   **Foundation:** Foundation is perfect for evening out skin tones and just like your concealer, yellow tones are best and the most natural looking.

★   **Powder:** You're gonna need a little of this to give your "base" some staying power and to resist shine through- out the day. Stay away from pasty white tones and opt for a color closest to your natural color. Apply with a *soft* brush (I personally love and will *only* use Trish McEvoy brushes) for a natural and soft look. Steer clear of those annoying puffs that are bound to make a mess in your vanity.

★   **Blush:** A blend is best. Make sure your blush gives you a hint of color, but not so much that you look like the Raggedy Ann doll your annoying aunt gave your unborn baby. Blend coral, pink, and plum tones with a more natural shade for a simply sweet look.

Hate to Admit It

The mask . . . well, they all said it would go away but like myself, my skin is STUBBORN and didn't let it disappear like so many of my friends' skin. My pregnancy mask turned into my postpartum mask! I still had the mask of pregnancy even two and a half years after my son was born! Well, here's the good news, there are products that can help fade the discoloration. (Triluma worked for me—ask your doctor about this topical cream AFTER you've had your baby and are done breast-feeding.) I tried everything and it slowly faded but I could always see the dark spots. I finally resorted to laser treatment, which worked wonders! And worked far quicker than the topical creams. If you can afford it and can tolerate the (minor) pain, I highly recommend talking to your dermatologist about this treatment. (Note . . . trust me, you won't even care about the "mask" after you see that beautiful baby you just created!)

Star Style: Jennie Garth

"You are supposed to glow when you're pregnant....Not always true! I sometimes enhanced my 'glow' with a slight shimmer blush on my cheeks. I love Cargo's Fresno. There is nothing wrong with a little help!"

—Jennie Garth, actress and mother of three

☀ REIN IN THE VEINS

Some rock star mommas report the appearance of little spider veins on their faces. You can pretty much bet their moms had them, too, since heredity plays a big part.

What generally happens is that blood volume and flow increases dramatically during your second trimester. As blood is pumped back to the heart, veins act as a one-way valve to prevent the blood from flowing backward. If that one-way valve becomes weak under pressure, some of the blood can leak back into the vein, collect there, become congested, and swell the vein. Because the veins are so close to the surface of your skin, they're easy to spot and, thanks to their jagged, spidery shape, look way more annoying than they actually are.

Two ways you can help prevent spider veins from appearing in the first place: 1) wear sunscreen, and 2) use a moisturizer that contains vitamin K, which appears to help clot blood just beneath the skin's surface and stop it from leaking back into the vein. Many vitamin K creams contain retinol, so don't even go there. One that doesn't, so it's safe to use, is Pharmaceris N Vita-Capilaril Active Moisturizing Cream. This super cream is a hydrating and replenishing cream that improves the functioning of the connective tissue. But once these spidery friends appear, there's little you can do (except reach for your new MAC concealer to camouflage them) until you've given birth. At that point, ask your derm about laser therapy or sclerotherapy if they don't disappear by themselves, which, *phew*, they probably will.

Just a quick FYI before you head off to the makeup counter: Those sudden hot flushes you've been fretting over? Annoying, yes, but they're just caused by those small blood vessels in your face rapidly fluctuating in size. No need to worry, just give a spritz of your facial water mist to beat the heat and return to cool you.

☀ EYES RIGHT

A word about your eyes. If you experience any eye trouble at all, chances are it'll be in your last trimester.

For instance, instead of waking up your usual, gorgeous rock star momma self, you may find your eyelids are puffy. Unless you were sobbing over a weepy movie the night before, it's nothing more than the effects of increased blood circulation. Bring down the swelling with slices of peeled cooled cucumber placed over each eyelid. (By the way, avoid all movies featuring kids or anything to do with kids while pregnant if you want to stay sane as well as gorgeous. And to be on the safe side, cut out animal-related movies, too.)

One of the most common eye problems is fluid retention, which can affect your eyesight if it puts extra pressure on the eyeball. Some women find they can't see as well when they're reading or doing detailed work. This fluid retention also desensitizes your eyes—which, strangely, is good and bad. You may find that your eyes aren't as aggravated when you put in contact lenses and you're able to keep them in longer than usual. Trouble is, the extra trauma on your eyes can result in pretty severe irritation and redness.

Sound familiar? Talk to your doctor. There's nothing I can recommend that's better than a pregnancy-safe prescription. But rest assured, your eye troubles will only be temporary.

ROCK STAR momma's Beauty Bag

You have the perfect excuse to go shopping. What are you waiting for—and what to buy NOW? Check out this handy list put together just for you:

- ★ Gentle facial exfoliator—AHA-free, please

- ★ Creamy face cleanser—to replace your skin-drying soap

- ★ Rosewater—instead of your regular harsh toner

- ★ Twenty-four-hour moisturizer, preferably one with vitamin K

- ★ Concealer—to cover blemishes, brown spots, and spider veins

- ★ Fragrance-free mascara—just one lash coat gives your entire face a lift

- ★ Lip balm—lips may be drier than usual, so you'll need a ready supply of balms. Avoid those containing camphor since it can be drying.

★ Lip gloss—a light sheer pink with just the right hint of color works wonders on all skin tones, and a girl can never have enough lip gloss!

★ Facial hydrating mist—travel-size sprays for extra tote-ability

YOUR HOT BOD

Now, I know you probably remember the day that puberty struck, right? Remember being a teenager when it seemed like every other day, something new had happened to your body . . . y'know, hips and thighs from nowhere, the sudden appearance of breasts and—yikes!—armpit fuzz that sprouts overnight . . . as well as hair down there!

Being pregnant is just like that, except in double time . . . actually, quadruple time! The way and speed at which your body changes is beautiful and exciting—it's like having front-row seats to the world's greatest miracle. And you are a miracle! But, girls, it's also a little scary and, you want the truth, downright freaky at times, too.

Your body will, for the first time in a long time, not feel like yours. And for many rock star mommas who like being in control of the way they look, and work hard to keep their bodies just so, it takes a while to get used to Mother Nature being in charge for a change. But she knows what she's doing. If you find you sweat more than usual or discover hair protruding from surprising places or strange marks on your skin, this isn't your body having a giggle at your expense. It's all happening for a very good reason . . .

So succumb to the pleasure of all the changes! Celebrate each new sign you're having a baby! Stroke your body, praise it, pamper it, nurture it, talk to it, tell it how much you love it. . . . In turn, you'll feel special, sparkling, sexy! Remember: This incredible journey lasts only nine months and enjoying it depends on how you embrace your new hot bod!

✳ WOW! IS THAT MY BODY?

Body Wow! #1: Your Blossoming Bod

Beauty Blah: Stretch Marks

Exciting telltale signs of pregnancy will start to show early in your second trimester (although second, third, or fourth pregnancies can show earlier). Your waist disappears, your midsection starts to swell, and breasts, thighs, and buttocks get fuller. But as your skin stretches in these areas, the connective tissues (collagen and elastin) start to tear and your body's forced to rapidly produce extra fibers to "glue" them back together. It's these extra fibers just beneath the skin's surface that show up as reddish/purple streaks we call stretch marks, and up to 80 percent of pregnant women get them. Whether you're likely to get them depends on three factors:

1. If your mom developed stretch marks when she was pregnant, chances are you will, too.

2. The paler your skin, the higher your risk of stretch marks. Darker skin produces more natural oil, which delays or prevents all sorts of skin nasties, from wrinkles to stretch marks.

3. The more you keep your skin hydrated and moisturized, the less chance you'll get stretch marks.

Rock Star Momma Solution

Some say stretch marks are pregnancy badges of honor. WHAT?! . . . NO WAY! Moisturize, moisturize, moisturize. Stock up on belly oils and creams (especially ones that contain vitamin E or cocoa butter, such as Belli's Elasticity Belly Oil, which has both and, thanks to lavender, also smells divine) and slather them on every night and everywhere from the moment you learn you're pregnant . . . if not before! Hey, I did this and there is NOT ONE single stretch mark on this body (don't hate me)! Plus, you've just gotta keep skin hydrated from the inside, too. So keep that Evian bottle close by and start guzzling!

Some mommas ask if you can ever get rid of stretch marks.

Well, the good thing is that it's never too late to start moisturizing. At the very least, it'll help those stretch marks fade more quickly once Junior's born. And if they still bother you six months later, ask your derm about retinoic acid, which can reduce the appearance of stretch marks by up to 20 percent. As a last resort, try laser treatments, which can be very effective, but—ouch!—it's expensive.

STRETCH MARK SOLUTIONS

"The number one skin concern of expectant mommas is stretch marks. In 80 percent of pregnant women, rapid stretching of the skin causes tears in the connective tissues that result in scars known as stretch marks (*striae gravidarum*). There is no proven way to completely prevent or erase these scars, but published research shows that daily use of gotu kola extract, vitamin E, and collagen hydrolysates help decrease their occurrence. Should you already have stretch marks, try a stretch mark minimizing cream that will help fade their appearance. Our cream features the research-proven ingredient darutoside—a plant derivative known for its powerful healing and regenerating effects. We recommend this product be used postpregnancy."

—ANNETTE RUBIN,
president and CEO of Belli Cosmetics

FROM A PRO

"Today's research shows that regular, deep hydration is the best defense against stretch marks. For centuries, women have used pure oils to moisturize, strengthen, and beautify the skin. During pregnancy, the needs of the skin change and intensify. We use a rich blend of high-quality oils including hazelnut, wheat germ, rosehip, grapeseed, and sweet almond oils plus vitamin E, selected for their complementary properties known to tone and regenerate skin. An oil blend works wonderfully because it doesn't sit on top of the skin feeling sticky; rather, it absorbs quickly to soothe itchiness and leaves skin feeling soft."

—KELLI KENNY AND LAUREN PARISIER,
cofounders of Basq

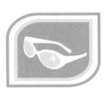

Star Secret: Kimora Lee Simmons

"I love beauty products, lotions, and smelling pretty and it was no different when I was pregnant, but the most important part of any pregnant woman's beauty regime is to moisturize, moisturize, moisturize! I cannot stress this enough! While some stretch marks are hormonal and hereditary, others can be prevented and you will feel much more comfortable."

warning

 Those same creams I just told you about could possibly stain your beautiful bed linens, so make sure you cover up that bod of yours after slathering on your favorite cream or oil. I know, it certainly doesn't sound sexy to hop into bed with your man wearing long johns and a sweatshirt, but it's just not worth destroying your favorite bedding.

Beauty Blah: Belly Itch

As hormones hare around your body and your skin is stretching so much to accommodate your growing baby, particularly in your second and third trimester, you can go insane with itching. It's called "pruritus gravidarum," which sounds pretty scary, but it just means "the itch of pregnancy" and it's nothing to worry about. In rare cases, itching is a symptom of a skin condition called prurigo, which looks and feels like a heat rash and is annoying but completely harmless. If the rash looks more like hives and you see it spreading, it could be **PUPPP**, which stands for **P**ruritic **U**rticarial **P**apules and **P**laques of **P**regnancy—because the bumps clump together in plaques. Again, nothing to worry about and your doctor can easily treat it. But it will go away on its own (promise!) when you deliver. In any case, if you are itching far more than normal or what you find tolerable, call your doctor!

Rock Star Momma Solution

It's the M word again. Is this getting boring? Too bad. I can't say enough about moisturizing for stopping stretch marks and itching and keeping your pregnant bod beautiful. Calamine lotion and cooling showers will also ease the itchies. Also try this: a cold milk compress. You won't believe how soothing this is. Turns out, milk is a natural anti-inflammatory, so it works wonders on itchy pregnancy skin.

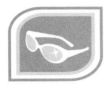

Star Secret: Mariska Hargitay

"The cure for an itchy belly is 'belly smooches.'"

Beauty Blah: Linea Nigra

Or the dark line of pregnancy that appears around the sixth or seventh month and starts at your belly button and travels down to your pubic hair. It's particularly obvious on dark-skinned mommas.

Rock Star Momma Solution

Nothing will stop this pigmentation. But rest assured—it will go away within a few months of giving birth. If you're self-conscious and worry it's showing through sheer clothes, simply wear thicker tops so you can be certain no one will see it.

DITCH THE ITCH

"Many women experience dry, itchy, and uncomfortable skin throughout their pregnancies. Regular exfoliation sloughs away dead, dry skin cells, allowing moisturizers and oils to penetrate more effectively. Next, try a cleansing body wash to gently clean and moisturize without stripping the skin of its natural oils. And most important, try a body lotion to replenish the moisture deep within the skin, leaving it silky smooth and positively radiant! A perfect way to pamper and comfort thirsty skin."

—ANNETTE RUBIN,
president and CEO of Belli Cosmetics

ESSENTIAL OILS TO AVOID

"While essential oils can provide great benefit during pregnancy, compounds in certain essential oils have emmenagogue properties (that is, they stimulate uterine muscles), which can have unwanted effects on the body during pregnancy. Other oils can be irritating to the skin and cause real discomfort. Women should always consult with their doctor before using essential oils and be sure to read the ingredient list of products they use during pregnancy. We performed extensive research of published work by leading aromatherapy experts. Experts publish lists of oils they believe are not recommended for use during pregnancy. Some examples:

angelica	myrrh	sassafras
chamomile	parsley seed	savin
cinnamon	pennyroyal	sweet fennel
clary sage	peppermint	sweet marjoram
ginger	rose	thuja
jasmine	rosemary	tansy
juniper	rue	wormwood"
mugwort	sage	

—KELLI KENNY AND LAUREN PARISIER,
cofounders of Basq

Beauty Blah: Outie Belly Button

It's not really a beauty blah, but some mommas aren't crazy in love with the way their belly buttons protrude in the later months of pregnancy. Kelly Ripa even says she received sackloads of mail from viewers *criticizing* her outie when she was heavily pregnant on *Live with Regis and Kelly.* I can't believe anyone would be offended by the natural, *normal* way one's navel sticks out due to the pressure of a growing baby. But if they are . . .

Rock Star Momma Solution

Tell them to get a life!! Honestly, anyone who criticizes you needs some volunteer work to put that pent-up energy to good use. But if, and only if, it's *you* that is uncomfortable with your new little accessory, nipple tape over your belly button will smooth it down under silky tops and dresses. Otherwise, flaunt that outie!!

Beauty Blah: Heavy Sweating

Hormones + increased circulation + all that extra padding around your torso = armpits like leaky taps. *Drip, drip, drip!* Fortunately, sweating is the way our clever body self-regulates its temperature. Unfortunately, it's not sexy and certainly doesn't do wonders for the ego when you can't stop the gross sweat stains under the armpits of your favorite silk blouse. So read on to help you both look and smell sweet.

Rock Star Momma Solution

Long-lasting, sweat-blocking antiperspirant is NOT the way to go. It's a lot savvier to wear layers of natural fibers so your skin can breathe and you can strip off easily as your temperature starts to climb. Take lots of cool showers to reduce head-to-toe body heat. And try a natural deodorant that won't block sweat ducts (sweating is healthy, remember!) but will keep you odor-free. You will love the Arbour crystal deodorant stones that somehow (no one really knows how) prevent whiffy bacteria from forming. One will last you all through your pregnancy.

Body Wow! #2: Beautiful Big Boobs

Beauty Blah: Breast Pain

If you always wanted bigger boobs, honey, you've got 'em now! For many rock star mommas-to-be, their swollen breasts are the first sign they're pregnant. So it's even more reason to celebrate—hooray! Trouble is, they're often tender and painful, too—booo! It's all thanks to hormones and dilating blood vessels, which are growing to nourish breast tissue and prepare for the development of milk ducts. The good news is that if your man can't keep his hands off your bulging beauties, he won't have to endure your screams of pain for long. By the end of the first trimester, you'll be taking just as much pleasure from your voluptuous new bod.

Rock Star Momma Solution

Upgrade to a bigger and better bra with wider straps for support and to ease muscle strain. A good cotton bra is best so skin can breathe, but there's no need to sacrifice sexiness and femininity. (A little lace goes a long way to make you feel like the vixen you are!) But, mommas, no underwire! At this stage, anything that presses into breast tissue will be painful. And later it could clog milk ducts. *Rock Star Momma* recommendation: Bella Materna bras. And finally, ensure your bra fits properly on the tightest row of hooks so you can wear it when you get . . . even bigger!

Beauty Blah: Skin Tags

Most likely caused by hormonal changes (what isn't?), small, soft, flesh-colored growths or flaps can appear anywhere on or around your breasts. You won't like them, but they're harmless.

Rock Star Momma Solution

Don't pick or flick. Just tell your doctor, who should be on the lookout for skin changes anyway, and he'll/she'll probably recommend laser therapy a few months after you've delivered.

Beauty Blah: Discoloration

Your breasts are preparing themselves for the use nature intended: feeding your baby. So as blood flow increases in preparation, your veins will become more visible, and the areolas—the pigmented circles around your nipples—will get darker and probably grow to the size of saucers!

Rock Star Momma Solution

A tan, or, better still, a *fake* tan, is the best way to camouflage dark-colored veins and feel a whole lot sexier. But stay clear of tanning beds, which can be dangerous

"If you are uncomfortable with a much-larger-than-usual chest, draw attention upward to your face with gorgeous oversize earrings and keep your neckline bare."
—ARIKA CHAN,
Arika C. Jewelry

to you and your unborn babe. Try dusting a *little* (repeat . . . LITTLE) bronzing powder to hide blemishes and veins. Just make sure to get the correct shade that will compliment your natural skin tone or you'll end up looking like the female equivalent of George Hamilton . . . yuck!

Body Wow! #3: Growing Gorgeous

Beauty Blah: Body Hair

You already know that your hair is growing thicker and faster. But—yikes!—that goes for body hair, too. As well as on your arms and legs, don't be surprised to see hairs sprout on your breasts, belly, and back (although, hopefully, it'll probably only be a few). And some women say they notice they get more hair on their chin, upper lip, and cheeks. Before you get busy with the jumbo tube of depilatory cream, read on . . .

Rock Star Momma Solution

Shaving, tweezing, electrolysis (only with your doc's approval), or waxing are the best ways to get rid of body and facial hair when you're pregnant. As your pregnancy progresses, I recommend booking an appointment with a professional to help take your skin back to hair-free smoothness, especially around the bikini area, where it's probably growing like grass but isn't so easy to reach after six months. But be warned! Your full-Brazilian wax may hurt more than usual, as pregnancy skin can be more sensitive, so just ask for a partial job. Don't risk anything that can be absorbed into your skin, such as bleach or depilatories. In any case, they stink so bad, they'll probably cause you to lose your lunch. *Ick.*

Beauty Blah: Never-ending Nails

You just had a manicure and, what do you know, your nails have grown another quarter inch already. What's going on? Hormones (of course!), which in some women cause finger- and toenails to grow at the speed of sound, and in others result in soft or brittle nails.

Rock Star Momma Solution

Keep nails fashionably short, squoval, and natural. And lose the fake nails. Those long, painted acrylics are so, so bad for your real nails and you really shouldn't be inhaling all that yuck during your pregnancy. The chemicals and sprays needed to apply them shouldn't be anywhere near you right now. I know, you love your manicures (who doesn't!), but I recommend you talk with your doctor about the potentially harmful ingredients in some nail polishes, such as phthalates and toluene. Both ingredients are suspected of presenting risks to reproduction and fetal development.

Keep hands moist with lots of hand creams, and if your nails are really brittle, try dabbing a Q-tip in baby oil and using it to massage your cuticles every day. And don't forget to wear protective gloves when you're washing dishes, using household cleaners, and gardening. Easy on the nails, good for the baby, too.

skin deep

I came across this extremely useful website in my research on nail polishes and their effect on pregnant women. Skin Deep (www.ewg.org/reports/skindeep2/) was developed by the Environmental Working Group, a non-profit research and advocacy organization focused on safeguarding public health. They have researched over 14,000 beauty products and provide safety ratings and detailed product ingredient information. This site is a great resource tool, but as always, first check in with your doc before heading to the manicurist (refer to the **Shopping Bag** chapter for more info on Skin Deep).

Beauty Blah: A Bigger Shoe Size

Pregnancy weight and a hormone called relaxin that loosens ligaments in the body (to open up the pelvis for childbirth) can cause your feet to get flatter and wider—and up to a half or full size larger. *No kidding.* In fact, up to 70 percent of rock star mommas genuinely have a great reason to go shoe shopping! Plus, feet can also swell thanks to water retention. Although those ligaments will tighten up postpartum and the swelling will go down, your feet may stay larger permanently—and may even increase another half size or more next pregnancy!

Rock Star Momma Solution

There's nothing you can do about your loosening ligaments and increasing foot size except to wear shoes that give excellent arch support. If that fails, grab a girlfriend and head for Jimmy Choo! As for your swelling, achy feet . . . a lavender foot bubble bath is gorgeous, but a foot rub from your man is even better.

Beauty Blah: Increasing Exhaustion

There are so many changes occurring in that lovely bod of yours, not to mention the extra little person you're carrying around (wow!). Backaches, headaches, swollen hands and feet, neck pain, stress, sore knees . . . sound familiar? Hardly surprising you're e-x-h-a-u-s-t-e-d. If only you could sleep properly . . .

Rock Star Momma Solution

When your doctor gives you the thumbs-up for prenatal massage (around the start of your second trimester), make that appointment and relax. Now is the time to pamper yourself and not feel guilty about it. Not for one minute! There are so many benefits, from better circulation to relief from aches and pains, it's the best beauty treat! Not only will you look and feel better, you'll sleep better, too.

Star Secret: Kimora Lee Simmons

"Try your best to stay cool, calm, and collected. Pamper yourself as often as you can—even simple things like taking time to put your feet up and read your favorite magazine or take a nap make a huge difference and will keep you focused on your fabulosity! My body changed so much! How didn't it change? Most changes I couldn't control, therefore it was important to me to still feel like myself. I continued to make an effort to be stylish, I continued my beauty regime, and prenatal massages didn't hurt, either! Pregnancy is an amazing time and there is no reason not to feel fabulous!"

sleepy sidenote

Try a maternity pillow for added comfort while sleeping or resting. They're carefully designed to support both your growing belly and aching lower back. Worth the fifty bucks or so? Definitely!

❊ PAMPER YOURSELF!

You're performing the most incredible, amazing, thrilling, miraculous task in the world. You deserve spoiling. Rock star momma, you deserve a treat—every day! Because if not now, *when?*

★ **Book a Manicure:** Ask them to shape and trim your nails. Bring your own polish to ensure it's supersafe. Go for the pretty pink polishes (with no harmful ingredients) from Honeybee Gardens.

★ **Plan a Girls' Day Out:** Go shopping, visit a museum or a gallery, get together for a picnic in the park.

★ **Get a Facial:** Choose one for sensitive, stressed skin.

★ **Go to the Movies:** Check out the latest romantic comedy so you laugh and cry. Either way, it gets rid of tension and you'll feel better!

★ **Splurge on Some New Makeup:** Good buys: pearlescent-tinted moisturizers; peach-toned blush and shadows for cheeks, eyelids, and forehead; rose-toned lip gloss. All give good glow.

★ **Pick Up a New CD:** Soft and relaxing or happy and upbeat. Music makes a rock star momma feel fabulous—and a good, loud sing-a-long is great exercise! Check out the **Shopping Bag** chapter for a list of favorites.

★ **Take a Nap:** If you can, why not? Sleep all you can now.

★ **Book a Hot Date with Your Man:** A delicious, candlelight dinner in the restaurant where you met or a walk on the beach under the stars. Or, hey, liven it up with a night at the comedy club—can you ever laugh too much?

★ **Join a Prenatal Yoga Class:** It's a terrific way to meet other rock star mommas and it'll also help you breathe and relax properly, as well as reduce swellings and aches.

★ **Get Your Eyebrows Shaped by a Pro:** It'll totally transform your face.

★ **Book a Blowout at the Salon:** Nothing beats great-looking hair.

★ **Buy a Fabulous Pair of New Shoes:** Even if your feet haven't grown, can a chick ever have too many shoes?

★ **Run a Warm Bath (Not Exceeding One Hundred Degrees):** Burn a candle of your favorite scent. I love lavender and vanilla scents, but your nose knows.

★ **Write a Letter to Your Mom:** Or your husband/partner, your unborn child, yourself! Buy some beautiful stationery and take time to reflect on these special days . . . and your hopes for your beautiful future.

below the belt

During the last trimester, you might experience physical discomfort due to your expanding uterus and weight gain. As your body continues to take over, your uterus presses on the diaphragm and stomach, causing shortness of breath, heartburn (ughh!), and indigestion. The hormone relaxin (yep, the same one that's causing your poor feet to grow along with the rest of your body) causes the pelvic joints to loosen in preparing for birth. Approximately one in every five hundred women is affected by a condition called symphysis pubis dysfunction, due to inflammation of the pelvic joint (are you having fun yet?). This causes severe pain in the pubic region or groin, and may also spread to your back or legs. Please call your doctor if any of these symptoms sound familiar and get checked out right away. You might also try a pelvic support belt for added support and relief.

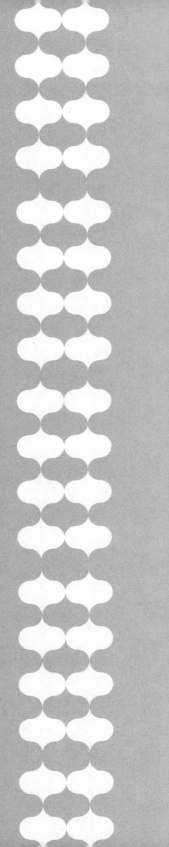

CHAPTER 5

dress-up *diva*

From baby showers to cocktail parties, rock concerts to formal functions, and let's not forget about those hot, sexy dates with your man, this Dress-up Diva chapter will help you look ravishingly radiant. Irrespective of where you live, whether you dress designer or discount (or both, now that it's the smart way to shop), and whether you're three months pregnant or nine, Dress-up Diva shows you how to find complete head-to-toe looks that fit, flatter, and feel *grrrrreat!*

Don't worry that you're suffering from style amnesia (did coral *ever* really go with powder blue, or anything else for that matter?). Don't fret that everything in your closet seems to belong to another person on another planet. Rock star momma, you've got enough on your mind. Just check out the following sections for the insider scoop on all things dress-up. I promise, whatever the occasion, Dress-up Diva's got you covered:

★ A Night on the Town

★ Black-tie Bling

★ Rock Concert Diva

★ A Date with Your Dude

★ Baby Shower Babe

★ A NIGHT ON THE TOWN

Even if they're not rollin' out the red carpet for you, they should be, thanks to the smokin' way you'll look in curve-hugging cocktail attire.

Think a vintage-inspired stretch-silk slip dress, a matte-jersey tube dress, a silk charmeuse halter dress in a bold, sassy print, a little black stretch-lace cami paired with the perfect A-line silk skirt. Each look offers always-flattering cuts in comfortable fabrics that'll help keep you smiling all night long (even when those shoes are killing your swollen feet and the little one happens to be resting on your sciatic nerve).

And let's not forget about accessories. Time to get serious

about sparkle . . . on ears, necks, and wrists. Sophisticated and elegant touches that ooze sex appeal with class and style. How to get it? Read on for tips on just how to paint the town red in this must-have get-dressed guide!

THE ROCK STAR momma's GUIDE TO A NIGHT ON THE TOWN

Where: WEDDING COCKTAILS

What to wear: Vintage-inspired stretch silk or breezy chiffon slip dress. Avoid to-the-navel plunging V-necks (attention should be on the bride, not your boobs!), but you can still dress up your décolletage with flattering ruching, ruffled Vs, or a neckline that's sensuously low and wide. Avoid big splotchy patterns; delicate and dainty is your desired effect.

What to wear it with: Hats are back, no kidding. Keep the vintage theme going with a wide-brim floppy hat, or, Sienna Miller or Jennifer Lopez–style you can throw in the air when vows are declared! Strappy sandals, a long, narrow clutch (for lip gloss, hydrating mist, and plenty of tissues), and swing it, sister, in the dazzle department: strings of necklaces (black pearls, loads of charms, semiprecious stones), bangles, and droplet earrings.

Where: NEW YEAR'S EVE FESTIVITIES

What to wear: Celebrate the start of a whole new year in a sexy strapless or halter dress. No need to stand on ceremony at this cocktail bash; just let your hair down and unapologetically

necklace chic

The perfect necklace can transform a simple sheath into a stunning outfit, take a sexy cami into an all-out fashion statement, and make over a boring top into something totally brilliant. Don't be afraid to be bold—go for numerous strands of differing lengths, big chunky beads, delicate charms, and more. Then mix them up to create an original look that's all yours.

cooler in color

Black, gunmetal gray, indigo, and chocolate brown are classic, beautiful, and cocktail party perfect, but when done right, a hint of fuchsia, garnet, red, or turquoise can be sexy—and certainly sassy. Don't be afraid to play with color. Start with baby steps and opt for bold colored jewelry, shoes, and bags.

flirt, flaunt, and fizz! However sexy you dress, make sure whatever lies next to your skin is soft, soft, soft—choose meltingly soft matte jersey, silk, or satin, fabrics that'll caress your skin well into the wee hours of the night.

What to wear it with: Nothing beats a pair of sexy stilettos with a strapless dress, especially when they're in a sizzlin' hot metallic . . . gold, silver, or bronze. Prints are in, too: leopard is a personal favorite, and so Versace couture! Balance those bangin' shoes with a simple black cocktail clutch (you know, the ones with the embellished/crystal closure). A New Year's Eve must!

Where: CHARITY EVENT OR BIG-TIME CORPORATE EVENT

What to wear: A simple, classy cotton jersey wrap dress is most appropriate. Thanks to the always chic Diane von Furstenberg, there's a reason why this style is still so fashionable thirty-five years after its birth! Yes, it was in 1972 when Diane first introduced the wrap dress!

What to wear it with: Gigantic rocks reek of bad taste here. Confine glitz to sophisticated solitaires with bejeweled kitten heels and a simple clutch.

Star Style: Gwyneth Paltrow

"It was evening wear that I found most difficult personally. I took a few pairs of nice trousers and had a tailor sew in big stretchy panels in the front that I wore with heels (low ones). My favorite top was a vintage kimono I bought in Japan. I had it shortened to about thigh length so it would cover my belly and I kept it closed with a nice pin. It was a nice evening look."

BLACK-TIE BLING

It's like there's a conspiracy: Even if you haven't been to a black-tie function in fifteen years, you can almost bet the farm that one will show up requesting your presence somewhere around your seventh month of pregnancy—and, momma, you gotta be prepared.

You see, for many, just the thought of a black-tie event invokes instant anxiety. Well, time out, desperate diva. The event is going to be a blast. You're going to look beautiful, no matter how pregnant that booty—and belly—may be. This section is here to help you figure out what you're going to wear. Stress-free.

ARE YOU READY FOR YOUR CLOSE-UP?

Three ways to ensure you look picture-perfect tonight:

1. Blow, Baby, Blow! **Sleek, shiny hair is a foolproof way to feel cocktail fabulous and camera ready. And thanks to all those hormones, your hair is probably thicker and lusher than ever (see chapter 4, Head-to-Toe Glow, for more on this). Blowing out your own hair is a test of Olympic-style gymnastics at the best of times; when heavily pregnant, it's practically impossible. So book an appointment with a pro. A good blowout will keep your locks looking hot for up to four days. Or just for the heck of it, ask your stylist to roll and set your hair in large, sixties-style curlers. Sarah Jessica started it . . . now you, rock star momma, claim this cocktail-cute look as your own!**

2. Lip Service: **When you flash your smile for the camera, make sure those pearly whites are bright! Best lip colors: red and pinks with a bluish tinge. Avoid orange and corals, which will give teeth a yellow hue when the camera's on you.**

3. Strike a Pose! **Photographs of this cocktail bash will be around for many years. Ensure you're remembered in the most flattering way, protruding belly and all, by making a forty-five-degree turn when the photographer approaches. Avoid straight on or sideways. You might try lifting your chin a touch and slightly tilting to one side to help combat those unsightly fat rolls you might be sporting just now in what used to be your neck region. Now, smile!**

✳ BRING ON THE BASICS

From Gwyneth to Brooke to Mariska to Rachel, and all you lovely mommas out there, I can tell you this . . . when it comes to black tie—whether it's for a wedding, red carpet event, or an extravagant holiday party—it's always best to be classically understated in your gown, focusing on fit, fabric, and flattery.

Only then should you bring out the black-tie bling to kick it up a notch. (Check out how Sarah Jessica Parker and Gwen Stefani did it in the Swipe Their Style chapter.)

How to find that perfect gown? Check it out:

★ Fab Fabrics: Embrace fabrics that are innately sexy yet subdued. Stretch silks, soft jerseys, sumptuous cottons, and delicate cashmeres are all great ways to go—and feel divine against your skin. Add extra sparkle with a slight smattering of hand-stitched beading.

★ Fantastic Fit: With a simple cut, it's crucial to have the right fit so that the dress flatters and feels good all night long. Thankfully, the "empire" cut is back and better than ever in the modern fashion world (if you want to sound swanky in the store, pronounce it the French way: "um*peer*"). Who can forget Heidi Klum in that stunning red gown or Kate Hudson wearing white

FROM A PRO

"My favorite fashion tip to pregnant clients dressing for a special occasion is to wear something sassy and comfortable. With the wide selection of maternity apparel available now, women don't have to choose the outfit that works or will do. Wear clothes that give you pep in your step and make you want to strut your stuff."

—SONG PARDUE,
CEO, Pickles and Ice Cream

Swipe Her Style: Gwyneth Paltrow

Hey, if they are good enough for Ms. Paltrow, then they'll be plenty good for you! Gwyneth was WAY ahead of the curve with the whole leggings/tights look. Truly, a look where function and style meet!

on the red carpet or Debra Messing in her utterly gorgeous Greek goddess–style gown. And Sarah Jessica Parker in her swingy, white empire-waist Narciso Rodriguez number. Or Rachel Weisz in an elegant-yet-simple black gown at the Oscars or the lovely Maggie Gyllenhaal at Cannes in her first big red-carpet event as a pregnant woman! And my personal favorite, Gwen Stefani strutting her stuff in *leopard*!

★ **Pretty Prints:** As long as you feel comfortable and confident in prints, then go for it. But, puh-leeze: no big polka dots or daisies, inky splotches, palm trees, parrots, or other cartoony creations. If fabric and fit are just right, a beautiful-yet-subdued print will help you make a sophisticated statement at any event. Remember Gwen Stefani's dress? If you can pull off leopard print like a true rock star, GO FOR IT!

★ **Bring on the Bling:** Jazz up a simply sophisticated dress with a fantastic, sparkling brooch, a chunky necklace, or a delicate diamond necklace. Bring your personality into your bling, baby, bling!

❋ SUCK IT UP

Now you've found a great dress for that formal wedding or black-tie ball, but you're feeling that booty is a little too jiggly for your comfort. What to do? Thankfully, there are fantastic undergarments out there to keep that jiggle from doing the wiggle. A one-piece body smoother is great for holding it all in place. The only trouble is that it can be a little bit . . . well . . . stuffy. Try the garment on for a few hours before the big night to get used to it. See the **Shopping Bag** chapter for where to get my favorite lifesaving line from Spanx.

That's it—that's all it takes to be a beautiful black-tie goddess! A simple dress, a little creativity, and the unwillingness to compromise on glamour, and you'll be the belle of any ball.

> "Rock star mommas wear Mama Spanx as an undergarment and a fashion accessory. When she was pregnant, married-to-a-rock-star Gwyneth Paltrow loved wearing our sheer black Mama Spanx footless pantyhose peeking out beneath the hemline of her dresses. She paired her Mama Spanx with a Calvin Klein dress and strappy sandals, when she was in Vegas for the ShoWest Awards."
>
> —SARA BLAKELY, founder of Spanx

ROCK CONCERT DIVA

There they are: tickets to U2. Or Coldplay. Or the Black Eyed Peas. Or any red-hot nighttime gig, for that matter. This is one event that calls for the ultimate in sexy, sassy, eclectic style—a look that's a little bit Goody Two-shoes *and* a little bit badass. Mixing up just the right amount of sweetness and spice to create a nighttime look that's almost too cool for school is, sometimes, just what the doctor ordered—especially when you're feeling so big, so pregnant, and so not cute.

Ready for this? . . . Think frayed jeans, a very vintage concert tee embellished in Swarovski crystals, and Dolce & Gabbana stilettos, with hair pulled back into a slick, sexy ponytail. Think must-have underbelly camouflage cargo pants mixed with a sexy black silk cami, knee-high boots, and an unforgettable cuff. Get it? Think looks that are inspired by fashion and music icons like Debbie Harry and Gwen Stefani. It's a look that just straight *rocks*.

DID YOU KNOW??

Gwen Stefani surprised her fans at a concert in Florida by announcing her pregnancy ON STAGE, shouting to the crowd, "Say it loud enough so the baby hears it," as they sang along to "Crash." In true rock star momma form!

Read on and check out the *Rock Star Momma* Get-Dressed Guide below:

★ **Star Shoes:** It's all in the shoes, they say, and I couldn't agree more. Shoes can make or break an outfit. Punk up even the most basic jeans and fitted T-shirt with some ankle boots or chic stilettos. From round-toe to a dangerously sharp-pointed toe, your shoes make a statement, even if YOU can't see your feet!!! Everyone else is looking!!

★ **Crazy for Cuffs:** This little accessory adds just the right amount of edge to any look. Whether it's a simple piece of leather or embellished with gold or silver studs, crystals, or other details, a great cuff can rough up any outfit in style.

★ **Tossin' On Tees:** I'm a little obsessed with the vintage tees, I admit, BUT they are just so comfortable and affordable and almost always look amazing! Always fashionable, try them on for day or night. How to make them transition to night? Dress 'em up, that's all. Wear with fitted jeans and knee-high motorcycle boots or wide-legged suit pants with a great pair of round-toed heels. Then bring on the jewelry—load up on the bangles and a pair of supersize earrings. You're rockin' it now!

glama-momma alternatives

If you're on a budget and your $$$ doesn't stretch to a gown, try these superflattering, starlicious substitutions:

• Black cigarette pants become nighttime worthy with a belly-hugging sparkly turtleneck and chic rhinestone earrings. Don't forget a metallic purse—find one cheap-n-chic at a chain like the Gap or Banana Republic.

• A curve-hugging pencil skirt and fitted blouse becomes viva la glam when you leave the blouse buttoned just to there and add big, badass earrings and a sexy skyscraper stiletto. An animal-print clutch is the purrr-fect accompaniment.

• A diaphanous wrap dress with spaghetti straps goes from demure to diva with a perfectly placed brooch that's bursting with pearls and crystals. *Ooooh,* and don't forget strappy sandals along with brightly polished toes!

beauty tip

When you want to go for all-out glamour, here are two bold beauty options:

• Break out the gold and silver . . . makeup, that is, but never together. Whether it's shimmer, liner, highlighter, eye shadow, or lip gloss, a touch of metallic makeup instantly gives sex appeal to black-tie glamour. Remember, everything in moderation, ladies!

• Smoke and mirrors . . . get gorgeously glam in a flash by going smoky. There's nothing sexier and it's so easy. Line your eyes with a dark charcoal gray or black liner and smudge softly. Then, apply a dark brown shadow on the lid—going right over the liner. Next add a lighter shade of brown with some serious shimmer over that darker brown on the inner parts of your lid. Finish with a crème highlighter under your brow and then blend, blend, blend. Layer on the black mascara—and if you're feeling it, even some individual fake lashes at the outside corners of your eyes. Smokin'!

★ **Deconstruct Me:** This look's not about nice and neat. More like supersassy and a little sweet, so aim for strategic deconstruction. From frayed edges to straight-up holes, a little bit of roughhousing can take any outfit from average to awesome. *Remember that cheese grater I mentioned earlier!*

Star Style: T-Boz

"When I was pregnant and had to dress up—when didn't I?—I'd choose to wear regular clothes in bigger sizes instead of those big ugly-ass maternity clothes. I shopped at Renaissance in Westlake, California, because their clothes were stylish and you could keep adjusting them as you got bigger."

—T-Boz, from TLC and owner of hip boutique Chase's Closet

A DATE WITH YOUR DUDE

Yes, there will be times in your pregnancy when you will inevitably burst into tears from exhaustion and pull out your hair with frustration at not being able to do the things you'd normally do (like sleep on your stomach, for instance! I know, pathetic, huh?).

But there's one thing you must have faith in . . . when your relationship's already good, getting pregnant makes it great. It's a terrific bonding experience between you and your beau. It's also when you start to realize that it may not always be just the two of you. Could well be three, four, five, or (yikes!) six of you down the road, who knows? So you'd better grab as much quality time together as you can. *Now.*

A date with your dude is a terrific opportunity to remind yourself and him—though it's my guess he doesn't need it—what a wonderful, unique individual you are. That as well as being a mass of hormones and a fountain of knowledge on every freaky birthing story known to womankind, you're also smart, funny, wise, sensitive, inquisitive, bold, brassy, and more. And you want a dress-up date look that reflects all that. A look that doesn't just ooze cool; a flirty, eclectic combo that's just right for night.

FROM A PRO

"Buy at least one dress that makes you look and feel fabulous. You will wear it to your shower, a friend's wedding, or on a night out with your sweetie. Women deserve to feel beautiful and look sexy during their pregnancy."

—SHANNON DiPADOVA,
founder of Due Maternity boutiques and website

fred flintstone feet

After a long day, those feet can sure get pretty darn swollen—especially if you're nearing the end of your pregnancy. Yet, for a look that simply rocks, it's just so hard to give up wearing those heels. To help shrink those feet back down to a size that can readily be semistuffed into a heel, take ten minutes out of your get-ready routine to just relax.

Put those heels up and apply a cold compress to those peds. The coolness helps constrict the swelling, while elevating your feet helps improve circulation, thus lessening the swelling.

You should also check out a great product by Modelco called Cool Feet Airbrush Catwalk Heels. Women swear by this miracle spray that instantly revives and rejuvenates sore, tired feet. Loaded with natural extracts of papaya (to revitalize), bamboo (to restore softness to your skin), chamomile (to relieve aches and pains), and peppermint (to stimulate), this is sure to be a treat for your feet. Refer to the **Shopping Bag** chapter for where to buy this fabulous creation.

Such as? A simple cotton stretch-jersey tube dress that goes from darling and daytime to dress-up delicious when you pair it with a jacket, a sexy necklace, and cool shoes. A vintage slip that instantly becomes an oh-so-hip dress when you throw a romantic cardigan over it. Pair it with some sexy shoes and a playful necklace and you've instantly reached hot-date status.

Need some more tips to help rev up the romance? Read on, lovebird:

ROCK STAR MOMMA'S GUIDE TO DATE DRESS-UP

★ **It's a Wrap:** Nab one of your favorite fitted nonmaternity tees and try it on. Is it too short? If you've popped, it probably is. Here's how to make it cool and the perfect pregnancy piece: Have your tailor sew on a Pucci-esque scarf along the bottom of the tee, leaving enough fabric to tie a loose bow on the side. Not only will it do the trick in adding that extra length, but you've just created a one-of-a-kind design, too. See, you're a couture momma now, too! No wonder he loves you . . .

★ **Lovely in Lace:** Lace is always good. Think Uma Thurman. Think Kate Hudson. A vintage-inspired lace cardigan over a ribbed tank top with jeans and heels screams "hot date" every time.

★ **Tube Tops ROCK:** A fitted tube top that accentuates your pregnant belly with a pair of wide-legged pants and stilettos is oh-so-sexy. Kick it up a notch by layering two tube tops. Two layers means double the support and an added color choice.

★ **Take the Plunge:** A plunging neckline can make you look like a million bucks—and ensure your sweetie adores you even more! (Not possible, but still . . .) For instance, a bohemian-inspired, butterfly-style chiffon top goes from hippie to hot when enhanced by a deep-plunging neckline to show off that sexy, new-found décolletage.

FROM A PRO

"I think it's essential that any mom-to-be not lose her sense of style, no matter what others may think. I had a funny incident when I was eight months pregnant with my son, Liam, and had just opened Naissance on Melrose. I had designed a sexy, leather halter maternity dress and I thought it was just fabulous. And, of course, I placed it in the window of my shop. Soon after, I found myself behind two women talking about my leather dress, making comments, such as 'Who would ever wear that?' And 'She's definitely going to go out of business.' I was horrified. But guess who went on to wear that dress? Jane Leeves and Jada Pinkett Smith. And you know what else? I'm still in business, baby!"

—JENNIFER NOONAN,
owner of Naissance on Melrose (NOM)

glow, baby, glow

A fresh, glowing natural look is always best, even at night. Babe, these forty weeks you're going to glow like you never did before, so you might as well enjoy it while you can! Rock the pouty-lip look with high-shine lip glosses, allow your eyes to shine with shades of shimmery shadows, and show off those cheekbones with a little bronzing powder and a hint of rosy blush applied only to the apples of your cheeks. Feminine and understated, just what the momma ordered!

✳ HOT DATE BEAUTY

Complete your date look with these in-the-know beauty tips, straight from the hip:

Berries and Cream: Every man I've ever met loves clean-looking fingernails, just buffed or coated with a dreamy, creamy natural polish. On feet, however, it's a different story. Toes look vampy and flirtatious with a sophisticated shade of berry. It's a beauty statement that goes from daytime to dress-up with ease. If you're worried about formaldehyde and toluene, opt for polish without—there are many polish manufacturers that offer formaldehyde- and toluene-free formulas. See page 114 in the **Head-to-Toe Glow** chapter for further nail know-how.

Touch-me Hair: Whether your hair is a cute crop or long and flowing, your beau will long to reach across the table and touch your tresses without losing his fingers in sticky gel, crunchy spray, or gloopy wax. If in doubt, keep it clean. Hair, that is. (What you talk about is between you two!)

The Scent of a Woman: Most mommas find their usual perfume too much to handle once they become pregnant. Yet, come the hot date, they feel underdressed without at least a small delicious spritz. My advice: Steer clear of complex fragrances from the big beauty companies (they're often packed with artificial chemicals, which can make you extra nauseous). Instead, go for simple spritzes of aromas you know you *both* love, such as grapefruit, lavender, orange, vanilla, or lime. I absolutely *adore* the scents from Comptoir Sud Pacifique (gotta try the Vanille Banane!), Jo Malone, and Fresh. I also really love the collection of perfumes from Serge Lutens, which uses essential oils and organic ingredients. The Un Bois Vanille scent is absolutely *divine*!

BABY SHOWER BABE

Well, baby—this one's for you (finally!). You're almost there. The last Big Event where the attention—and those cameras—are still all about you, because you know that any and all attention focused on you ends the second Junior makes his appearance, right? So, of course, the pressure is on to look *gorgeous*. Yep, whether it's a girls' brunch at your favorite restaurant, a family shindig at Aunt Beth's house, or a couples' barbecue at your best pal's clubhouse, you've just got to look good. Those pictures are sticking with you for the rest of your life, so you will want to look like the radiant rock star momma you are. Simply put, those pix are going down in history.

The trouble comes built-in, of course. Most baby showers happen between months seven and nine, when you're likely as big as a house, things are feeling snug, and you're so sick of every single thing that's hanging in your closet. So what's a gal to do? Don't stress. Just follow these easy do's

Sometimes there is nothing better than a few moments of peace and quiet before heading out to a big function. Taking a few deep breaths, focusing on healing pressure points, and breathing in doctor-approved essential oils can be just what the doctor ordered to rejuvenate, revive, and refresh for your big night out.

and don'ts to help get you started (and as always, go with your instinct . . . only you know when you feel your absolute best!).

DO wear something comfortable, yet memorable. You're going to be looking at those pix for years to come and you don't want to look like how you may be feeling, now, do you?

DON'T wear something overly loud or trendy—remember, this one is going down in picture history. That's not to say you can't get creative—just tone it down a tiny, tiny bit, that's all. Simple is always better.

DO wear something that highlights your assets. Got boobs? Tastefully flaunt them with a simple V-neck wrap dress. Buff biceps? A graceful sheath will do the trick. Hot legs? A sassy mini is just calling your name . . . if you dare!

DON'T wear something that looks majorly matronly, however comfortable it is. Now is a good time to invest in a cute, fitted, and flattering maternity dress or form-fitting top you can wear with looser pants. Other suggestions: a favorite body-hugging tee and a long, languid skirt, or a gorgeous blazer over a tank top and jeans. These types of looks will make you look slimmest on film.

DO wear something that makes you feel like a million bucks. Stick to colors that make you look radiant, fabrics that feel good (baby-soft cashmere or merino, mercerized cotton, breezy linen), and cuts that you typically gravitate toward.

Today isn't the day to experiment with a new look, even if your hormones are telling you otherwise.

DON'T play dress-up if that's not your schtick. For example, if you're a jeans kind of girl, then wear them. You can deck out the rest of your outfit to pull off jeans with panache, honest.

THE ROCK STAR MOMMA'S GUIDE TO SWANKY SHOWER STYLE

Need more help in finding the perfect outfit for your special shower day? Just read on to check out these insider tips for looking simply swanky at your shower. But please, dress for yourself as well as the event. This is *your* time:

★ **Sundress Sistah:** You just can't go wrong with a sundress—it's always fresh, always in style. Better yet, if you can wear a strapless sundress, then do so—it's sexy and sophisticated all in one. Opt for a halter top or empire line. If it's on the chilly side, throw on a cropped cardigan knit—looks adorable tied under your boobs. Thank God the capelet and every reincarnation of the design is still going strong, as this piece works wonders!

★ **Dress You Up:** Few dresses are as easy, graceful, and polished as a wrap dress, thanks to Diane von Furstenberg. (No wonder she sold five million in the first

hair help

A subtle pony, a tousled wave, or sleek and straight are ideal shower dos. None are too trendy, while each is equally pretty, soft, and romantic. Just be sure to tame any frizzies and flyaways with a light grooming crème. If hair is misbehaving—or even if it isn't, and you just want a do that's chic and off your face—turn to the band! Suddenly they're back in style and made from all sorts of lush fabrics from raffia to silk, butter-soft leather, and chiffon. So, so easy to add a touch of style and sophistication to any shower look.

color me beautiful

If you're feeling sassy, try vibrant jewel-tone shades of ruby, emerald, amethyst, and sapphire. Dresses and blouses in these tones are best in soft, subtle fabrics with very little sheen.

four years of designing them!) In supersoft jersey, with pearls and a pair of kitten heels and hair tossed into a loose bun, you've got a pristine shower look that would make anyone proud.

★   **Bohemian Belle:** A peasant-inspired top with dressy capris and heels or a long, layered, romantic skirt with a belly-hugging top are both always stylish, especially when your shower is a Sunday brunch. Kimono-cut tunics are always flattering, too.

★   **Totally Tubular:** Pair a tube top with a layered skirt or cargos and a chunky necklace for a delicate yet rockin' outfit that's perfectly memorable and easy to wear. Remember, comfort is key!

★   **All Suited Up:** A great suit is always an appropriate choice for any baby shower, especially if you've got a beautiful cami underneath to show off that belly. Classy. Sassy. Sophisticated. Shower-worthy.

There you have it: As long as you stay true to your fashion comfort zone, you'll feel—and look—like a million bucks at your shower, even if you *are* feeling big as a house!

the last word

Whatever the event may be, remember that your inner beauty and confidence are what make any rock star momma radiate. Dressing up helps us all feel extra-special. Just remember that no matter how pregnant you are, how gross you are feeling, how fat you may feel, you are a beautiful mother-to-be! Just that thought alone should give you the comfort and confidence to pull off any look with joie de vivre.

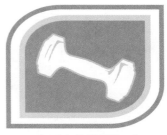

gym *goddess*

Staying fit during your pregnancy encourages a healthier baby, an easier delivery, and a quicker recovery. In fact, the pros say that working out can shorten your delivery time by up to two hours. Hey, if there is anything that evokes even the thought of an easier time pushing Junior out, I say go for it. And, of course, there's the added obvious bonus: Working out helps with the whole weight gain thing. So needless to say, it's a great idea to make fitness a key part of your pregnancy lifestyle. A word of caution, though: You've got to clear any exercise plan with your doctor before getting started.

While a well-rounded fitness and well-being program is an important element of a healthy pregnancy, looking good in

yoga momma

With your doctor's okay, yoga is an ideal form of exercise to practice throughout your entire pregnancy. Taking regular yoga classes helps increase physical strength, mental relaxation, and blood flow and oxygen to the uterus. Many RSMs find that regular yoga also helps reduce swelling, back and leg pain, and insomnia. Most important, yoga is a great way to connect with your growing baby. Ommmn . . .

workout gear isn't always as easy as it should be. Think you can pull off an old T-shirt and some oversize sweats and call it workout gear? Think again, rock star momma. Gone are those baggy tees and paneled pants—they're just not part of your maternity wardrobe. Rather, enter Gym Goddess: a smart, savvy, sexy you who takes pride in how she looks—even at the gym.

How to be a Gym Goddess? Just use this chapter as a guide for finding exercise wear that looks and feels great during the many stages and sizes of pregnancy. Whether it's for yoga, Pilates, weights, or simply out for a walk with your man, through the following sections, you'll have more than enough info on how to be a fabulously fashion-fit momma-to-be:

★   Bras with Bragging Rights

★   Rockin' Tops

★   Hot Pants

★   Sneaker Pimps

A WORD FROM THE WISE

 During pregnancy, there are many changes a woman's body goes through. It is important for a woman to understand these changes so she knows how to safely modify her exercise routine. Fitness during pregnancy is now considered an essential part of a woman's prenatal care so she will have a healthy pregnancy, an easy labor, and a faster recovery. Important tips when exercising:

- Do not get overheated.
- When doing aerobic exercise, control the intensity by making sure you are always able to carry on a conversation.
- Drink at least eight 8-ounce glasses of water per day. Drink more if you are exercising.
- Do not do exercises and activities that put you at risk for falling and abdominal trauma (e.g., back-lying exercises, skiing, Rollerblading, horseback riding).
- Do upper-body exercises in a seated position. Motionless standing can cause pregnant women to become light-headed and dizzy.
- If you become light-headed or dizzy when doing exercises in a back-lying position, roll to the side to get the weight of the uterus off the major blood vessel it might be constricting.
- Do not do regular crunches or crossover oblique exercises, as they make the separation of the abdominal muscles larger.
- When working with weights or Dyna-Bands, do slow, controlled movements with muscle, not momentum, moving muscle. Avoid jerky movements. Pregnant women's joints are looser and they are more at risk for injury.

—JULIE TUPLER, RN, certified childbirth educator/certified fitness instructor, National Council on Strength and Fitness

BRAS WITH BRAGGING RIGHTS

It's *très importante* to invest in supportive bras during your pregnancy. Remember the advice I gave you back in **Panty Shmanty**? Max out on support now to prevent sagging later. When you're exercising, this holds true more than ever—you just don't want those boobs to bounce all around—so it's time to invest in some well-fitted, super-supportive athletic bras, bras with serious bragging rights for keeping your boobs right where they belong.

Yes, you might have heard that some gals wear two regular sports bras at once rather than investing in the real deal. Now, you're smart enough to figure out that your breasts need extra-special TLC right now, not strangling and suffocating.

When it comes to sports bras, you've got plenty of choices, but the amount of support you need depends on the type of activity you're going to be doing. For instance, power walking on the treadmill certainly calls for a bra that provides a lot more lift and hold than the bra you'd wear while striking a warrior pose during prenatal yoga.

Use this Sports Bra Shopping Checklist as a guide to finding the right one for you:

The Checklist

✓ **Fit:** As with your regular bras, your sports bra needs to have the right fit. You'll want the bra to stay in place, so try it on before you buy, and don't be afraid to perform some experimental stretches in the dressing room for a minute or so. It should neither ride up nor slide around. But make sure the under-the-boob band doesn't dig into your skin, either, which can happen as your rib cage expands or you retain water. Avoid ugly (sorry, but it is) back bulge by ensuring your bra's cut high under the arms.

✓ **Fabric:** Comfortable, stay-dry fabrics are essential. When you're six months pregnant and dragging your tired ass to the gym, the last thing you want to deal with is an itchy, uncomfortable athletic bra that retains sweat. Rather, go for fabrics that pull moisture away from your skin so it can breathe better. High-compression polyamides and cotton/Lycra mixes keep you dry and comfy, and reduce the risk of rashes and irritation. They tend to be a tad more expensive but are definitely worth it!

✓ **Support:** Fortunately, there are loads of sports bras from a plethora of manufacturers—from Nike and Adidas to Mothers in Motion (theirs are especially awesome for big-boobed girls), Spanx, and Danskin—that are all about serious support. You've got it right when you jog or power walk and your boobs don't do "the bounce." A great supportive bra will keep them in place so that the only bouncing going on is from you shaking your booty to the rhythm of your iPod.

✓   **Hooks:** This is about comfort and personal preference. Instead of the traditional nonadjustable band that many sports bras offer, quite a few manufacturers are now boasting supremely supportive bras with adjustable hooks and straps—some that even hook in the front, which makes them a great transitional bra for nursing. Try on a full array with different hooks so that you can find what's most comfortable—surprisingly, what was perfect for the pre-pregnancy you may be a complete turn-off now.

ROCKIN' TOPS

Today's workout tops are all about funkin' it up, while being functional, cool, and comfortable. Be sexy and play with bright, bold colors, prints, and styles—you just can't go wrong. And no matter what the style, make sure that your workout top is made from breathable fabrics, because it's critical that you don't overheat—it's bad for both you and baby.

Talking of which, make sure you gulp down a ton of water before, during, and after your workout. You've just gotta replace fluids frequently when you're exercising, since pregnant women have a tendency to dehydrate more rapidly. Plus, drinking lots of water will help you stay cool.

THE HiP GiRL'S GUIDE TO WORKOUT TOPS THAT ROCK

In case you just can't figure it out on your own, here's a handy guide to finding athletic tops that are just plain cool:

★ **Fit:** No matter how far along you are, make an oath right now and declare those ultra-loose, tentlike maternity tops to be official fashion faux pas. Rather, load up on workout tanks and tees that show off your blossoming bump with a fitted look. You'll not only look hot, you'll feel more comfortable without all of that loose fabric draped around your midsection.

★ **Built-ins:** So many workout tops have built-in bras, which are a great thing—but only if they offer the support you need. Remember, moving boobs + exercise + pregnancy = major drooping. Better be on the safe side and double up with an athletic bra underneath.

★ **Layering:** Rock star mommas love the layered look. Nothing's hotter than two tank tops layered just right, so naturally this holds true for when you're working out, too. As long as you're comfy, cool, and dry, work

help wanted

Need extra breast support at night, especially during that first trimester when even so much as the sight of a regular full-support bra can cause searing boob pain? Sleep in a sports bra! It's comfy enough for sleeping and supportive enough to make sure that those boobs stay put, which helps with the "ouch" factor. Later in your pregnancy when your breasts are at their biggest, sleeping in a sports bra will help prevent skin stretching and development of the dreaded stretch marks.

those layers for a look that's especially great in both those beginning months, when you're feeling mushy, and those end months, when you're feeling like the Goodyear blimp.

KEGEL MANIA

Listen, girls, there's something you have to know. Yoga's terrific for poise and flexibility, and nothing works your little heart out better than walking, cycling, and swimming. But if you want to facilitate an easier delivery (hello, who doesn't?), emerge from this pregnancy with your perineum (that delicate area between your vagina and anus) intact, and safeguard your sex life after your baby's born, you'd better start the Kegels. Oh, and did I mention, it prevents incontinence, too.

Not sure what Kegels are? Next time you go to the bathroom to pee, try stopping and starting the flow. The muscles you're squeezing to stop peeing are what's called your "pelvic floor" and the purpose of Kegel exercises is to get them nice and tight.

The basis of a Kegel exercise is the squeeze-and-hold. So, rock star momma, when you're chilling on the treadmill, squeeze in a few sets of them. Squeeze and hold—two-three-four-five-six-seven-eight-nine-ten . . . or for as long as you can. Believe me, the more you do, the better they work.

Course, you don't have to be at the gym to do your Kegels—you can squeeze and hold in the car, in line at the grocery store, while brushing your teeth, watching TV . . . even while you're making love (betcha he'll feel the difference!). Keep on Kegel-ing right up until you deliver—it may get more difficult as pressure from the baby increases, but it's still having a positive effect on that all-important pelvic floor.

Alrighty, now that you've got your top half covered, let's check out those hot pants.

HOT PANTS

✓ WHAT'S HOT?

When it comes to those workout bottoms, comfortable, sexy, and cool is totally hot (sorry, all you Paris haters . . . I know, she ruined a perfectly good word for all of us!). Think about showing off those curves in form-fitting workout pants with a flare or bootleg cut. Feeling leggy? Try running shorts that show off your toned getaway sticks (if you've got 'em). Is sassy more your style? Then toss on flared capris in a bright, bold color. *That's* hot.

✓ WHAT'S NOT?

Skintight spandex leggings have never been your friend, nor will they ever be—not even in this seemingly qualifying time of partial desperation. Just *fuhgeddaboudit*. That is, unless you're lucky enough to look like Heidi Klum . . . God bless you!

✓ HOW TO GET HOT?

Ideally, your workout bottoms should have great fit, flatter even your not-so-flattering parts, and provide a divine amount of comfort. And, if you feel like a hot momma, chances are you'll be less inclined to bail out on exercising. Well, you'll have one less excuse, anyway.

flat out

Never exercise flat on your back after the fourth month— it's just downright dangerous for your baby's development. Why? According to the American College of Obstetricians and Gynecologists, any kind of exercising on your back compresses the inferior vena cava blood vessel, which is responsible for getting blood and oxygen to the baby. That goes for ab work, too.

✓ WORD TO THE WAISTBAND

Rock star mommas are all about finding the perfect mix of comfort and style. That said, an under-the-belly style is always best for working out. Wear with a fitted tank, a great sports bra, and some sassy sneakers, and you're ready to take on the world.

If you're a runner, however, under-the-belly waistbands won't do the trick for you. For you running mommas, it's all about maximum support. Go for an over-the-belly fit made from fabric that keeps moisture and heat away from your skin.

✓ FITNESS FLASH

Here's a quickie chart to help you find the best workout pants for an array of exercises for all nine months . . . and even beyond:

YOUR EXERCISE:	WEAR THESE BOTTOMS:
Walking	Drawstring trackpants; under-the-belly flared, boot-cut, or capri leggings; under-the-belly walking or running shorts.
*Running**	Over-the-belly waistband with built-in support; fitted, slight flare, or straight-leg styles in breathable fabrics to avoid tripping.

*Spinning**	Under-the-belly-waistband shorts or capris with built-in tushie padding; if pants, straight leg is best to avoid snagging in pedals.
Prenatal Pilates	Flare, boot-cut, or capri bottoms that allow for movement and keep you cool; under-the-belly styles are best.
Prenatal Yoga	Comfy, double-deep yoga pants or loose-fitting under-the-belly drawstring pants that allow for movement and flexibility.
*Weight room**	Stay-cool, breathable pants that allow for movement in an under-the-belly waistband and flare or boot-cut legs.

---

* Don't even think of doing this form of exercise without checking first with your doctor—no matter how cute your workout pants are!

gym do

Hair got you in a tiff? Nothing is cuter—and easier—than donning a cool hat and ponytail at the gym. If hair's long enough, braid it. Keep bangs from sticking to your forehead with the help of a colorful headband or some rhinestone hair clips.

SNEAKER PIMPS

Cool sneaks can make even the simplest workout gear look ultra-fabulous, while giving you the proper support and comfort that those peds deserve, especially since those feet can change so much during pregnancy. From increased sensitivity to yo-yo swelling, they sure can be unpredictable. So *walk this way* . . .

Check out the Sneaker Pimp Survival Guide to find the perfect workout shoes for your pregnancy:

★   Fit: Has it happened to you yet? When those feet grow a half to full size during pregnancy? When those perfect sixes morph into sevens? Nines become tens and tens teeter on elevens? If it hasn't, you may be one of the lucky few whose feet don't grow . . . or, it may be lurking around the corner. The same hormones that are working on loosening up the ligaments in your body to prepare for childbirth may also cause your feet to grow longer—and spread wider! Take no chances with ill-fitting sneaks—go and get measured. Once you assess your true size, try on a few pairs and dish out the dough for a pair of new kicks. And get over the size thing quick—you're just as cute as an eleven!

★   Straps: The chances that your feet are going to swell are pretty darn high, especially while you're working out. Velcro or other loose ties will allow you to quickly ease tension as they increase in size.

★ **Comfort:** Your feet—and your joints—are a lot more sensitive during pregnancy. As those hormones loosen up your ligaments, you're more prone to aches and pains, so it's extra important to have great support and a cushy, shock-absorbing foot bed, especially if you're into walking or running.

★ **Traction:** Who knew that sometime around month six, all of that coordination and grace that you worked an entire lifetime to perfect were to be tossed out the window? For some of you, right around this time Super Klutz enters and Graceful Goddess goes on hiatus. So you want to be extra careful when you're working out— those moves you once had down in your sleep can suddenly become, well, grace-impaired and may be placing you at risk for accidents. Why the change? All that extra weight in your belly can cause you to lose your sense of balance. Skid-resistant soles with a lot of traction are the way to go to help minimize any chance of pregnancy-induced, grace-impaired accidents.

★ **Color:** Play with bold colors and fun styles to add just the right amount of je ne sais quoi to your athletic wardrobe. Thankfully, the latest crop of quality athletic footwear is far more stylish than ever before. Bold colors such as orange, aqua, and yellow can now be

the stripe

What's up with "the stripe"? You know, the ones that so many athletic manufacturers stitch down the side of the leg? I LOVE this stripe! It magically breaks things up and helps the world see a trimmer version of you, and who can complain about that? And the same goes for vertical panels on workout tops—contrasting baby blue or white between two black panels elongates your bod and looks supersleek and fit.

seen on cross-training styles, allowing your fashion sense to never be compromised, even at the gym or Pilates class! Get funky, baby.

✳ GYM GIRL TO GLAM GIRL

Go from Gym Girl to Glam Girl in five minutes flat. First up, toss that hair right back into a sexy, disheveled ponytail or loose bun. Next, apply a thin layer of moisturizer to your face, followed by stick foundation to help cover any unevenness, like the mask of pregnancy or a hormonally driven blemish. Brush on some loose powder to set and then follow with a light concealer—just a quick swipe under the eyes is perfect. Next, use an all-in-one bronzing stick as blush and shadow—it'll brighten you up, especially if you're feeling pasty. Finish with mascara and some seriously sheer pink lip gloss—it's just the best color for making everyone look pretty, restored, and revived. That's it! You're out the door, momma, and you look fabulous!

the last word

⭐ Working out is great for the mind, body, soul, *and* your baby. Looking good while you're doing it is good for *you*. Embrace this time and pamper yourself with exercise gear that makes you look and feel good because you deserve it, rock star momma!

hospital *hip*

Nope, it's not a weekend away at your favorite Four Seasons or Ritz-Carlton, but you're about to head off to create the most exciting, beautiful, and amazing miracle. You're about to bring life into this world, so shouldn't you look good while you're doing it? Especially since you've made it this far in your pregnancy, embracing a style that totally rocks.

As long as you're prepared, it's actually pretty easy to look great while in the hospital or birthing center or wherever else you may be heading off to deliver your precious cargo. The key word, of course, is "prepared." Don't worry—even you die-hard procrastinators will be able to get it together with a bit of help from this section.

In this chapter, you'll learn what really needs to be packed (warm socks) and what doesn't (blow-dryer, anyone?), as well as what you're really going to need for baby—both at the hospital and for that trip home. Plus, check out the many handy checklists to help even the most disorganized gal get ready for the Big Day with ease—from writing your contact lists to devising your birthing plan.

And don't forget to take care of Dad—after all, he's half the reason you're heading off to that delivery room, so he sure deserves to get some special attention, too. Well, that and the very strong possibility that your inner Linda Blair, a la *The Exorcist*, may come out in the delivery room. My bet is that if and when your head starts spinning, you'd want your man to be nice and buttered up to help him better deal and not hold it against you for days, months, or (gasp!) years to come. So, in the pages ahead, be sure to pay attention to the must-have guide to hookin' him up in the delivery room.

There's also some straight-talkin' style advice for going home, since you probably can't even think that far ahead right now. The truth is when you come out of the hospital with your beautiful newborn, you'll never see the world the same way again—and you'll want to record that joyful journey, looking radiant and gorgeous.

Hospital Hip is loaded with the ins-n-outs to show you how to dress accordingly. Check it out . . .

- ★   Labor Loot

- ★   Daddy Gear

- ★   Baby Booty

- ★   Homecoming Queen

LABOR LOOT

So you're almost there—somewhere around thirty-two weeks in. The light at the end of the tunnel is rapidly approaching and hopefully all that's left to do are the finishing touches on the nursery. You've completed every birthing and Lamaze class under the sun and are even having dreams of tennis balls, controlled breathing, and whirlpool tubs on a regular basis. You are getting ready to make that major transition from rock star momma-to-be to straight-up rock star momma. And in doing so, there are bags to be packed, checklists to be tended to, things to get in order.

Take my advice: **Pack early.** You just never know when that stork is going to make its appearance and most times, it's no-where near where or when you thought it would be. It's like he's got his own clock that pays no attention to yours or your doctor's.

First stop? Time to get organized and get the almighty list together of what needs to be done. And don't fret, it's not so bad. Keep reading, it gets easier . . .

The Get-Ready-to-Go Checklist

✓ **Pre-register at Your Hospital:** Do it as early as you can; it'll save you much time and effort on the Big Day—if you're having contractions, the last thing you're going to want to be doing is sitting in the hospital lobby filling out endless amounts of paperwork. Get any and all other hospital-related paperwork together, as well, including your insurance card, and stick them in a folder.

✓ **Little Black Book:** Get together a master list of important contacts, phone numbers, e-mails, and addresses. Then, break it down into four lists:

1. The Emergency List: Include your doctor's number, the hospital's main number, the doula's, any key relatives or friends who are going to join you for your labor, any neighbors that you need to feed or walk the dog, and so on.

2. The Call List: This is the list of names and numbers of those you'll need to call from the hospital when baby makes his or her appearance. Don't omit those names and numbers that seem like no-brainers, like your parents or grandparents. Even if you've had their phone numbers memorized since you were three years old, delivering a baby does crazy things to your brain and you may actually forget it in the moment.

3. *The E-mail List:* This is the list of those who you'll send a mass e-mail to announcing the baby's name, delivery time, weight, length, and, of course, baby and momma's health. Create the e-mail ahead of time, filling all of those addresses in well in advance and saving the message as a draft. Then, when baby comes, just have Daddy fill in the blanks and hit send. *Ta-da!*

4. *The Baby Announcement List:* This is the list of those who you'll send your totally chic announcements to. Once baby comes, you're going to be all-encompassed with him and are going to be glad this is done. It'll make addressing those envelopes so much easier later. (In fact, you really should address those envelopes NOW while you have the extra time.)

AVOIDING ANNOUNCEMENT ANGST

"Do yourself a favor and confirm every detail of your birth announcement several weeks before your due date—the design, the typeface, the ink color, and the wording. When you do give birth, you will be able to simply call in your baby's specs to your stationer. Also, ask your stationer if you can get the envelopes printed earlier. This way, you can really prepare before your baby's birth, while you have the time, by addressing and stamping all the envelopes."

—WANDA WEN,
founder of Soolip

✓ **The Master Plan:** If you are using a birthing plan, get it together as early as possible—that way, you'll be relaxed and ready to go on the Big Day. Well, as relaxed as you can be, anyway!

✓ **Work It:** If you're a workin' it woman, be sure to talk to your human resources department early on. There is more than likely a ton of paperwork for you to fill out for both your firm and the state, so get it out of the way.

✓ **Bind It Up:** Now stick all of the information that you've collected from above into a handy folder. When you get ready to pack your bag, simply toss this baby in there so that you have all of this info right at your fingertips.

STATIONERY SMARTS

"The announcements and thank-you notes you choose have become an extension of your personal style. Stationery has become a fashion statement just like the jeans you wear or handbag you carry. The motifs, colors, fonts, and paper you select for your stationery reveal your individual personality. Always order more stationery than you think you need! We are constantly working with frantic moms who urgently need more announcements or thank-you notes!"
—MATTHEW GRENBY AND IRENE CHEN,
cofounders of iomoi

Now that you've got "the list" in place, it's time to get that bag packed! This is, no doubt, the most exciting trip you'll ever make. Really, where else do you head in as two and leave as three . . . or more?

Following is the Rock Star Momma's Must-Have List for all things hospital hip to help make your trip as comfortable and stylish as can be. Note: I've intentionally left out stuff for baby, because it truly deserves its own section, which, if you keep reading, you'll get to. Check it out—and then *get packing!*

THE ROCK STAR MOMMA'S LIST FOR HOSPITAL HIP

Here's what to pack for the most comfort and style during your labor and delivery:

★ **Loungin' Around:** While you're chilling at the Hospital Inn, might as well look and feel cute. Excellent loungewear = cotton tees/tops with drawstring beach/pajama pants, or a darling cotton cami paired with velour or terry trackpants, especially if it's got a built-in bra. Plus, it's easy access for breast-feeding after delivery, which is key.

★ **Nightgown:** Think *black.* Why? Girl, you're having a baby. Yes, it's miraculous, but it's also messy, and if you're going the vaginal route, you'll be in a seemingly

pampered princess

A friendly reminder to keep those toes looking good—especially from here on out. Make sure you're waxed/tweezed, colored, scrubbed, and polished—try to keep up on all that beauty maintenance . . . not only do you want to look good at the hospital, but it may be a long time after baby is born before you can pamper yourself again, so get it all taken care of now.

car seat safety

Purchase your baby's car seat *early.* Actually, if you have the luxury, buy two. Keep one either in Daddy's car or in the garage so that Grandma, Grandpa, Aunt, Uncle, Nanny—whomever—can readily have access to it without you having to always take it out of your own car.

car seat style

And what better way to bring your beautiful new baby home than in an adorable infant car seat cover by Monica Rodgers! Let's face it, you can do better than that dull, generic car seat. Monica created a line of car seat covers in bright colors, soft fabrics, and classic retro prints. And best of all, these universal-fit covers are durable, washable, and extremely hip and cool! Check out the **Shopping Bag** chapter for all the shopping info you'll need!

permanent state of menstruation for the next six weeks. A black cotton sliplike nightie is just perfect for looking cute and feeling comfortable, while offering easy access for breast-feeding, too. Need I say more?

★ **Granny Panties:** See above note. That means maxipad mania for you, dear momma. Leave the hot G-strings at home—they won't make an appearance for at least six weeks. Choose those granny panties in dark, super-breathable cotton.

★ **Maxipads:** The hospital will keep you stashed on maxis; however, they are truly hideous and uncomfortable. Stock up on very absorbent pads—you will thank me later.

★ **The Fuzz Factor:** There is nothing more cushy, luxurious, and wonderful than a superlush robe to curl up in before and after delivering your bundle of joy. Check out the **Shopping Bag** chapter in the back of the book for the best of the best.

★ **Socks, Slippers, and Slides:** You just never know how you're going to feel when you get into the nitty-gritty of labor. You may not want to leave your bed or you may feel like you want to walk around the block to help ease the pains of those contractions. In case you do, be prepared and pack some extra-cushy socks (I just love those high-tech socks with added traction on the soles) and slippers. Plus, after your bundle of joy arrives, you'll want to have those slippers close by for those bathroom runs. And, then, why not a cute pair of slides or flip-flops that make you smile and you can easily slip on and off?

★ **Nursing Stuff:** Let me start out by saying that your milk might not actually come in for a few days after your baby is born. With that said, you may already be home, but it's better to be prepared for whatever might happen (like an unexpected C-section). In the "normal" course of events, your baby's sucking stimulates your body to make prolactin, the hormone that produces milk. Prior to the arrival of breast milk—and let me tell you, you will definitely know when this happens, as your boobs will suddenly take on a life of their own!—your body produces colostrum. This special milk is extremely easy to digest and contains antibodies to help keep your new little one healthy in the first few days of life. The more often you feed your baby in the first two to three days, the quicker your milk will come in. Regular feeding also helps prevent engorgement. . . . *Ouch!* And if you decide not to breast-feed, let your doctor know in advance so you can be well prepared for the changes your body (and boobs!) will go

car seat

Once you purchase your car seat, have it installed right away by a pro. Just contact your local police station to make an appointment for them to do so for you—most communities have several officers on staff that are trained to properly install the seat while showing you how to do it on your own. Scary fact: A DaimlerChrysler survey found that although 96 percent of parents believed they had installed their child's car seat correctly, fewer than 20 percent had! Give yourself giant peace of mind knowing that your little peanut will be going on his first car trip in the safest ride possible. And remember, the hospital will not let you go home without that car seat installed.

planned babyhood

So you're having a C-section or your labor is being induced. One good thing . . . you can plan ahead now that you know "the date." Lucky for you, you know the day, time, and minute you will have that baby of yours, so you have a slight advantage over other mommas-to-be. Get packin', girl, and for once in your life, don't wait till the last minute!

through to stop the production of breast milk. Now, as I was saying, it's important to bring along a few key items to get you started:

✓ **Cotton Nursing Bra:** As your milk comes in, you're going to want to be wearing a bra—it's just more comfortable to do so. For more details on nursing bras, visit the **Panty Shmanty** chapter!

✓ **Lanolin Cream:** Just trust me on this one. Your nipples will thank you. Remember the sucking part I just mentioned?

✓ **Nursing Pads:** Yup, your boobs are going to leak. Depending on how long you actually stay in the hospital, you might not need to bring these lovely accessories with you. But play it safe and pack a few just in case.

★ **Toiletries and Makeup:** Pack an overnight kit with the essentials—shampoo, conditioner, brush, soap, deodorant, toothbrush, toothpaste, lotion, shine serum, concealer, blush stick, lip gloss, and mascara. If you're a shiny gal, toss in some powder, too. That's all you need to get picture-perfect ready, hospital-hip style.

✻ SOMETHING SPECIAL

I just love this idea. Spend the afternoon with your mom or your man and together go and pick out that special outfit you'll wear while delivering your baby. Look for something comfy, cozy, and loungy. Trust me, you might have a lot of time in the hospital to walk around and girl, no one—and I mean NOBODY—needs to see your icky old jammies! BedHead pajamas are a rock star momma's favorite, as they are bright, cheery, and so incredibly comfortable. Make sure you look for lightweight cotton button-down styles since you'll need accessibility to all your private parts at any given moment. I also recommend long-sleeve versions since hospitals tend to crank up the AC! I think every woman needs something like that . . . whether it be a fresh pair of pajamas or a new robe or new T-shirt—you need that something bright and PRETTY. And you'll have that lasting memory of spending the afternoon with that someone special (your mom, mother-in-law, husband, or even your older son or daughter).

hospital hair survival

Leave the dryer at home. Seriously. You are so not going to feel like doing the full-on blowout after pushing out a child. If you've had a C-section, well, now you're really over that blowout idea, anyway. If your hair is long enough, a loose bun is pretty and practical. And a sleek pony is a winner, too. Just pack a light shine serum to tame any unruly pieces, that's all.

GOWN GLAMOUR

"While laboring at the hospital, my doctor saw me and said, 'You look too good to be in labor.' I refused to wear the nasty, homely hospital gown—I needed all the strength I could muster for delivering a baby, and the hospital gown was going to suck the life out of me (read: hospital gowns are not available in cosmetic colors, not to mention the open-air fan in the back!). So I insisted I wear my own garments and delivered my little one in our sexy nursing dress. Talk about delivering in style!"

—ANNE DIAMOND,
cofounder of Bella Materna

Tote Number Two

Now that you've packed those critical pieces that'll keep you cute and comfortable, organize a second tote that'll up the pleasure quotient of your hospital hiatus:

✓ *Snack Attack:* **Labor** can be a long, long process. And a girl's got to eat. So pack a bunch of snacks to keep that tummy content. Or you can always send a relative out for whatever food you (and Daddy!) might be craving— you've made it this far being so good, why not go out with a bang? Indulge, momma!

✓ *Read All About It:* **Bring** along some of your favorite mags to help pass the time. Or get back into that novel you've been meaning to finish.

✓   *The Film:* Don't forget to pack up your camera and videocamera. Even though it sounds like an easy given, I had to mention it. While you're at it, pack a backup camera, too—a cheapie disposable with a flash will do the trick. Be sure to charge your batteries and if you do have an extra battery pack, bring it along.

✓   *All You Need Is Music:* Pack your iPod and travel speakers so that you can rock out to whatever suits your taste during your labor. Make a "Birth Day" playlist with your faves ahead of time so you've got tunes at your fingertips.

GREAT ADVICE!

"For moms and dads—even at the fanciest hospitals, moms and dads *must* cozy up the atmosphere. Bring a little cheap low-wattage lamp, some candles (if allowed), and hours and hours and hours of mellow music! Try ambient Brian Eno! For babe—bring your own mini skullcap so when he or she is wheeled away to the nursery, he or she won't look like all the other babies! And for dads—moms, don't forget about your mate! The hospital blankets given out will leave them shivering at night. So have the new pop bring warm pajamas or an extra blanket."

—PAULINA QUINTANA,
of Paulina Quintana

the av effect

The effect of audio and visual stimulation during labor is, simply put, *amazing.* A meaningful picture or familiar film can truly help take you to another place as you make your way through heavy contractions. A favorite song can calm your nerves and instill a slower, steadier heartbeat. Whether you aim to go for an au naturel labor or an epidural, embrace the AV effect no matter what. Besides the calming physiological effects, there's nothing like adding a familiar comfort to an unfamiliar situation, and using pictures and other images and music are truly an easy and effective way to do so.

✓ *Massage Madness:* Toss in a massage lotion that smells divine. Sometimes there is nothing better in labor than a great foot, hand, or back massage and it sure helps to have your favorite lotion on hand.

✓ *Hair Stuff:* Bring some barrettes, hair bands, and headbands with you; it can get pretty darn warm during labor and . . . well . . . a little sweaty.

✓ *Journal:* You're going to have some down time, so why not write a little bit in your baby journal as you're actually going through your labor?

DADDY GEAR

Well, the time has come and your little one is en route to making that grand appearance. More than likely, even though daddy-to-be is acting oh-so-cool, inside he's pretty much freaking out. Whether it's that giant epidural needle or the idea of blood and stuff happening *down there* or just the crazy notion of meeting his offspring for the first time, there's no doubt he's needing some TLC to make him feel okay right about now. And since you're a little busy getting ready to push out that baby, my bet is that you just might be fresh out of TLC to share. My suggestion? Hook it up well in advance. Get together a special kit for your man—just sneak it into your suitcase and surprise him with it when you get to your room. Some things to include:

★ **Game Boy:** Pack a portable gaming device, like a Sony PSP or Nintendo Game Boy DS, with a couple cool games to help pass the time. The PSP is capable of playing movies, too, so visit amazon.com and click away for some cool flicks. And if you don't have the PSP, then . . .

★ **Movie Buff:** Pick up a little portable DVD player, along with a few of his favorite movies if you have the room, to help keep him—and you—entertained. Some hospitals now have DVD players (and flatscreens!) in the labor and delivery rooms, so you just might be in luck. I suggest calling in advance to avoid lugging any unnecessary stuff to the hospital.

★ **Man Mags:** Hook him up with some reading material that he'd actually be into. Leave parenting mags in your own bag—there'll be plenty of time for planting such valuable reading later!

★ **Sturdy Snacks:** Whether it's Doritos, cookies, Snickers, or the all-time guy favorite, beef jerky, toss in some of his favorite treats for him to nibble on to help pass the time. A man with a full belly is a happy man, and that's just what you want.

★ **The Mush Factor:** Stick in a handwritten card in which you share your feelings about this exciting time in your lives. When our hormones are in overdrive (which they will be for weeks, maybe months, yet), it can be difficult to express heartfelt sentiments without dissolving into buckets of tears.

That's it—it just takes a few little thoughtful things to help make your man more at ease during your hospital adventure. And if you follow the Daddy Gear guide, you'll make him not only happy, but relaxed. And there is nothing better than a relaxed man in a time of need.

BABY BOOTY

Packing for Junior's entrance into the world need not be as complicated as it's made out to be. You're not moving into the hospital, just temporarily visiting. The fact remains that babies require stuff. Check out this list for bringing everything you'll need at the hospital for baby:

The Rock Star Baby Booty Checklist

✓ **Hello, World:** Pack a memorable outfit for bringing your little one home—it's a major photo op that will forever go down in history. Better yet, pack two or three—you just never know when your beautiful bundle is going to spit up and need to be changed. Pick up something cute and appropriate that's all about easy access (i.e., a Communion-inspired dress is so not cool for this occasion). Obviously you want it to be cute for pix—this day is going down in picture history—but also make it easy to manipulate. Make the getting-dressed stuff as painless as possible.

✓ **T-shirts:** Side-tie T-shirts are easiest for getting on and off and make cleaning the baby's belly button really simple (which you'll do until the umbilical stump falls off). But some mommas like onesies, T-shirts that fasten under the crotch to prevent it from rolling up baby's back. Up to you, but pack a few.

✓ **Sleepers and Sacks:** Two or three of these are just enough to keep your newborn cozy and cute while chilling with Mommy, Daddy, and all of those fabulous new faces.

✓ **Receiving Blankets:** You'll want to bring receiving blankets for swaddling baby. Take my advice: A swaddled baby (in other words, one that's wrapped tightly like a little silkworm) is a happy baby. Since he feels protected, he'll sleep better, too. The hospital's receiving blankets are certainly not the most fashionable, but they ROCK. Why? They are longer than most and are the perfect size for comfortably swaddling. Get friendly with a nurse and ask her for the hookup! But remember, these blankets are hot commodity items, so don't be surprised if she doesn't give 'em up on the first try.

✓ **Spit-up Cloths:** These cotton cloths, placed over your shoulder, take care of that other new phenomenon in your life: spit-up. It's just something that pretty much all babies do after feeding. Grab a six-pack.

✓ **Jacket:** Bring along a jacket that's appropriate for your climate. Then get baby all bundled up before you head out into the world. That said, don't be an overbundler, some-

LITTLE ANGEL

"When shopping for bodysuits and one-pieces for your newborn, get touchy-feely with the fabric—pull them out of the packaging if necessary! It's all about comfort: wrap-styling is definitely the most gentle to wear and easiest to put on. And always choose 100 percent cotton—your baby deserves the softest textures on her precious new skin!"

—EMILY MEYER,
creative director of Tea Collection

thing that many first-timers tend to do. For instance, if you're in Tucson in the middle of summer, there's no need to bundle! Dress the baby as you dress yourself.

✓ Accessories

★ **Hip Hats:** A baby's heat escapes through his head. Regulate his internal temperature with a unique cap that also helps him stand out in the hospital nursery.

★ **Fab Feet:** Socks also help him keep warm when he's in nothing but his T-shirt. Forgo booties at this stage—plenty of time for baby Nikes later . . . it's all about comfort.

★ **Soft Mitts:** Babies tend to bat at their face with those little hands and it's amazing how sharp their nails can be. Pack a couple pairs of baby mitts to prevent uncomfortable and unsightly scratches. You can get them at any baby store or pharmacy—no need for anything fancy.

★ **Hair Bows:** Have a little princess on your hands? You never know if she's going to come out with a full head of hair. For the sake of pix, you may want to pack some cute bows to clip her hair with. Might as well start the diva training young, right?

★ **Diapers and Wipes:** The hospital may send you home with a few, but just in case they don't, better safe than sorry. Fragrance-free, please!

all washed out

Stock up on Dreft (or any mild, scent-free baby detergent) and prewash all Junior's clothing well in advance. It'll make life much, much easier when he makes his grand entry—especially because, for the next year, you'll be doing endless loads of laundry!

HOMECOMING QUEEN

Time to think about going home. Truth is, it doesn't take that much planning, since most maternity clothes are made in shapes and soft stretchy fabrics that look and feel good both before and after the birth. All you really have to decide is what'll look best on you as you stride happily through the door with your precious cargo (there's bound to be someone photographing you!).

THE ROCK STAR MOMMA'S GUIDE TO PERFECT HOMECOMING DUDS

Can't decide what to wear? Check out these cute combos that are sure to rock the house:

★ **Tracksuit Momma:** Think about some cute velour or terry trackpants. Slip on a soft-next-to-your-skin tissue tee and you're good to go.

★ **Cargo Cool:** Some low-rider khakis are perfect for your homecoming—always flattering. Simply pair up with an empire-waisted smock top to conceal that probably loose belly.

★ **It's All in the Jacket:** Jackets are your new best friend—they hide those love handles and those extra pounds in both your arms and that tummy. Wear with low-waisted pants for an easy look that rocks. Too bulky? Try a poncho. Perfect for draping over any size tummy.

★   Call It Like It Is: Toss on one of those kitschy "Just Had Baby," "Got Milk?" or "New Momma" tees to just call it like it is. Cute with a low-waisted floral skirt and sandals!

★   Button Up: Button-up blouses are perfect for concealing that "just-had-a-baby" stomach. Add a newsboy cap and some low-rider cargos for a homecoming outfit that simply oozes style and comfort.

★   Accessorize: Add some oversize hoop earrings and some hip tennies and you'll make an entrance that's casual, cool, and completely rock star momma.

☀ REALITY CHECK

Keep in mind that even after you've delivered that gorgeous baby, you will still look pretty darn pregnant. Go easy on yourself, momma. It takes time—between six and eight weeks—for that uterus to contract and your belly to go back down, even if you've only put on twenty-five pounds. Breast-feeding will certainly help shrink your uterus and whittle the extra weight away. But there's a reason for the saying, Nine months on, nine months off. In other words, if it takes that time to grow this huge, it'll take that time to get back to normal. Actually, it sounds a bit depressing. Heed this advice: Don't compare

coming-home tip

After being in the hospital for two to five days, you'll probably have that gross hospital smell all over your body, especially in your hair. If you feel up to it, and if you have help around the house and can sneak away for thirty minutes, a shower will do you wonders! That first shower at home...OH MY GOSH! You have NO IDEA how fantastic that will be! I promise, you're going to feel like those women in the shampoo commercials where they look like they are having way too much fun in the shower—need I say more? Hey, it's not every day you introduce your new little one to the world, so do whatever it takes to look and feel as good as you should!

yourself to the celebrities you see all over the newsstands. Remember, they have a whole army of personal trainers and nutritionists solely focused on squeezing their clients back into their red-carpet gowns as soon as possible.

With the proper discipline, exercise, and not too many all-out food feasts, you just might be able to get back into your favorite jeans within three to four months. Just don't expect, mere hours after giving birth, to be lounging in an outfit that boasts your pre-pregnancy size. It's not going to happen. And if it does? Well, count your blessings, because you are one of the very few postpregnancy body miracles. (And yes, I am completely envious. Don't ya just hate Heidi Klum???)

∅ NO, NO, NO!

Don't even *think about* packing these in your suitcase:

- ✗ **Pre-pregnancy Jeans:** Don't spoil this happy event trying to squeeze yourself into your favorite Sevens. They're just not going to fit right now. Accept it now and move on.

- ✗ **Any Pre-pregnancy Fitted Tees:** For the first time in many, many months you're going to want to hide that belly, so loose is best.

- ✗ **Anything Too Body Hugging:** Best to minimize those bulges, not call attention to them. They'll go away in time—I promise. *Nine months up, nine months down.*

PICTURE PERFECT

"For new moms, a gold locket on a long chain makes the perfect day or night accessory—it's superchic and is an easy way to carry a tiny picture of your little one with you at all times."
—ARIKA CHAN,
Arika C. Jewelry

✗ **Anything Dressy:** While you want to look cute, there is no need to get decked out to go home. Pass on the slip dresses and stilettos.

congratulations!

⭐ YOU. DID. IT!!! Style, grace, confidence, and life helped you be the ultimate rock star momma—not to mention a little bit of planning mixed with a touch of luck.

Now it's time to get ready for the ride of your life—MOMMA-HOOD! As you head into this new chapter of your life, always keep close at heart the feelings you now have about this grand accomplishment. It'll give you inner strength, peace, and a confidence like no other—you created the most amazing gift: LIFE. How cool is that? Keep that confidence in your pocket always, and much like a good-luck charm, it'll be by your side, helping you to tackle anything that comes your way.

You are—officially—a true rock star momma!

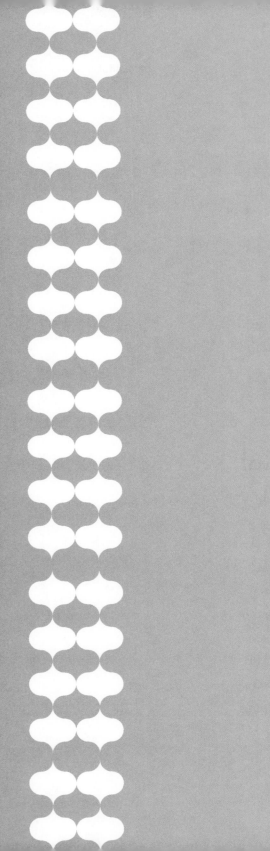

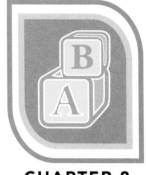

postpartum
panache

ou've made it—you're now a new rock star momma! Somewhere in between the seemingly endless feedings, the burpings, and the changings, you're bound to realize that a girl's still gotta get dressed. After all, you've gotta look your best in all those photo ops! Right? And, well . . . unless by some lucky stroke of God you're already back into your old clothes, most of us are still dreaming about the day when we can squeeze back into our favorite True Religions!

First off, don't stress on it . . . you *will* get there. In the meantime, what-oh-what is a girl to do? Postpartum Panache is here to help you. Whether you've put on twenty-five pounds or seventy (remember me, fifty-plus!! Yikes!), this chapter will help you get comfortable, flattering, functional, and ultra-hip style for this transitional time.

Besides the dish on looking hot during this fashionably funky time, there's also the essential guide to finding great nursing tops that offer easy access *and* style simultaneously. They *do* exist! You just need to know where to find them. It's all ahead . . .

And, *Rock Star Momma*'s also got the scoop on cool diaper bags, because much as it pains you to put your favorite Balenciaga bag on the shelf, it's just got to be done. For now. Because not only isn't it big enough for all the stuff that goes with your baby, but for the next year, you're going to want to carry a bag that is strong, sturdy, and won't break your heart if it gets a little beaten up.

For all of this and more, check out the following sections in Postpartum Panache!

- ★   Nursing Nice

- ★   Transition Tops

- ★   Bring on the Bottoms

- ★   Bag Lady

- ★   Rock Star Daddy Diaper Bags

NURSING NICE

If you're breast-feeding, you've not only got the postpregnancy wardrobe to deal with in the weight department, you've also got to make sure whatever you don has easy access. Just imagine this: You're out to lunch with your girlfriends and Junior is starting to purr for *his* lunch—Mommy's milk. Yet, the shirt you have on is SO not boob-friendly, meaning you've practically got to take it off come feeding time. Thus, you must excuse yourself to the ladies' room, cop a squat in a chair—if you're lucky—or worse, on the toilet (good God!), just so that you can feed your little one. Uh-uh, that's just not going to cut it for a rock star momma and her rock star baby.

Wouldn't it be so much easier for you, your baby, and your friends to enlist the help of an easy-access nursing top (that are now much more stylish than EVER before!)? Combine that with a strategically placed blanket or scarf over the chest and voilà! You can actually enjoy lunch with the ladies again!

So, now you've got to find some nursing tops that rock! The fact is you don't need to dress in traditional "nursing" tops to make breast-feeding a breeze—you just need to know what to look for in regular tops to help accommodate your ever-changing breast size while providing easy accessibility. Fortunately, there are now some pretty amazing lingerie lines out there to help you look gorgeous while nursing your little one.

☀ THE BEST OF THE BEST

Is there any woman sexier than Elle Macpherson? Nope! I mean, did you happen to see the 2006 *Sports Illustrated* swimsuit issue? It's hard to imagine that that woman is a mother of two! As I mentioned earlier in the **Panty Shmanty** chapter, Elle currently offers two gorgeous nursing bras in her collection: the La Mere and the Maternelle.

Star Style: Elle Macpherson

"This nursing bra (the Maternelle) is my absolute favorite item for moms and I believe every new mom should have one. The best thing about this bra is it's sexy, it fits well, it's supportive, and it's pretty and comfortable. Congratulations and happy bonding with your baby. Here's to the sexy mom in all of you!"

—*Elle Macpherson*, Elle Macpherson Intimates Collection

Another line that new moms are talking about is called Bella Materna. They have a built-in shelf bra that you can open up for breast-feeding by using just one hand. *Awesome!* And it's made from an amazing Italian Lycra-and-nylon mix so it keeps moisture from sitting next to your skin (dampness causes irritation). A word of advice: It's not so good for DDs. But for everyone else, this tank is so perfect, you would never know it's a nursing top.

And you have to check out the nursing tops by Majamas, especially their reverse cami. It's a three-quarter top that looks like you have a tank on underneath. When you start to feed, you simply pull the tank aside and your breasts are easily accessible, just peeking through these holes, still supported and so easy. (See the **Shopping Bag** chapter for more on this great company.)

For more rockin' tips to help you make the most of this boob-a-liscious time—whether you're going to nurse for two months, six, a year, or beyond—read on for the essential Guide to Nursing Tops That Rock!

THE ROCK STAR MOMMA'S GUIDE TO NURSING TOPS THAT ROCK!

★ **Easy Access:** Need I say more?

★ **Shapely Shirts:** As your breasts fill up with milk, they're obviously going to get bigger, so you want a shirt with stretch to accommodate your swelling bosom. And, once they're emptied, your top should have memory—that is, it should readily move with you as your breasts expand and contract. There's nothing worse than a top that looks stretched out and saggy.

★ **Bra-rific:** Make sure your nursing tops afford you the ability to wear a nursing bra. You'll not only want the support of a great nursing or sports bra to help keep

relax don't do it.

Ah, those first few weeks of baby bliss can be more like baby boot camp. How's a girl to survive? Take a deep breath. Roll with the punches. You managed to create this life, and you can certainly take care of it. You can do it. How? Ask for help. The most successful people in the world will tell you that they aren't afraid to ask for help when they need it, so you should, too. Ask your mom to do the laundry for you. Hire a night nurse for two nights a week. Have your best friend bring you dinner. When there's a new baby in town, people come out of the woodwork to see him and to offer their help to Momma. Take it. You—and your baby—will be so glad that you did.

sleepwalker

Are you feeling it yet? Exhaustion. The type of fatigue that has you functioning in a constant state that feels way too close to sleepwalking? It gets better. Promise. Sooner or later, baby will sleep, and when that magical night happens, oh boy . . . your face will respond with an instant makeover. In the meantime, how to cover those dark circles and bags to at least give the illusion of a well-rested you? First, use a hydrating eye cream to moisturize those tired eyes. Then, using your fingertips, apply a light concealer to cover any circles. Finish with my all-time favorite, Yves Saint Laurent Touche Éclat, to add a light-reflecting effect that will make even the most sleep-deprived momma look like a well-rested beauty.

you from sagging (with all of that swelling and contracting going on, now it's more important than ever to give those breasts tons-o-support), but you'll also want a good bra to help prevent leakage, as well. Line your bra with disposable breast pads and change them often. For more on nursing bras, visit the **Panty Shmanty** chapter for Nursing Bras 101.

★ **All Buttoned Up:** Button-up blouses are a great way to go for nursing. They can be a little oversize to compensate for those pounds that still need to come off, while still looking cool, as long as the rest of your outfit is tailored and sleek.

★ **It's a Wrap:** Wrap tops and dresses are fabulous for nursing! They offer great access and are truly flattering on any build. Stick to prints to help you look slimmer—and camouflage any milk stains. (Yep, I said milk stains!)

It's that easy to find nursing tops that rock. Just a little creativity and an unwillingness to compromise on convenience is all you really need. Keep the same qualifications in mind for nighty-night time, as well. When it's 3:00 a.m. and you're in a sleep-slash-breast-feeding haze, you'll want to have a nightgown or cami that provides comfortable accessibility for your little guy or gal, as well.

❋ DON'T FORGET: *CONVENIENCE*

Remember, you are now operating heavy pieces of machinery (those would be your boobs!), which might feel somewhat foreign at first, but trust me, you WILL get used to them and the best piece of advice I can offer is to make it as easy as possible to be able to feed your baby when he or she is hungry. And you don't have to sacrifice your sense of style . . . stretchy tanks, classy striped button-downs, and a quality nursing bra is a must-do combo for any nursing momma.

TRANSITION TOPS

If breast-feeding isn't your bag, no worries—that's a personal choice and who can't respect that? You've still got to get dressed and you've actually got one advantage over your nursing friends: after you get past the rather uncomfortable process of having your milk dry up, you don't have to give a second thought to those boobs. So you've got a lot more options when it comes to transition tops. Check out these handy-dandy tips below for finding great tops for this transitional time that will help hide and flatter those trouble spots:

★   **Lovin' Loose:** Up until now, I've pretty much shunned the idea of you ever wearing a looser top. The thing is, up until now you were pregnant and had a beautiful belly to show off. Now, rock star momma, you've got a belly that you want to get rid of. That'll happen soon enough. But in the meantime, a little bit of loose is just what the doctor ordered to cover it up. Just pair with fitted pants to help even out the look, okay?

★ **Just Jackets:** A jacket over a tank top, a T-shirt, or a tube top is a great way to help conceal that curvaceous midsection. Just button one or two buttons right across the middle of your tummy to help cover up that bulge.

★ **Tracksuit Couture:** Tracksuit jackets are still your friend—and they always will be! Zip up with a bold-colored tracksuit jacket over jeans, a loose and long skirt, cargos, trackpants . . . just about anything to create a comfortably cool look that'll help hide your newfound trouble spots.

★ **Smock Tops:** Tops with smocking can be very flattering and helpful in covering up that belly. Plus, in a bright, fun terry it can kick up any outfit from boring to brilliant!

BRING ON THE BOTTOMS

Ah, the joys of motherhood: puke-stained clothing, sleepless nights, burp-filled days, curdled milk in your hair, and a belly that just won't budge fast enough. But when you look at your angel and see the sparkle in his or her eye, that smile on his or her face, and that look of innocent curiosity all around, suddenly it all becomes worth it. Why did you have to try to squeeze into your old Sevens?

Never fear—you will get there. Remind yourself yet again that you've just had a baby. A BABY! Honestly, it just takes time, and until your doctor gives you the green light to exercise, just accept that it is what it is. If you're breast-feeding, it's likely to come off quicker, since your body is hard at work burning calories. But nonetheless, it still takes around eight weeks to see anything resembling your pre-pregnancy tummy and butt.

In the interim, check out these must-have tips to finding bottoms that fit, flatter, and feel great—no matter how many extra pounds you may be a-packing.

★   **Low Riders:** Once again, low riders are making an appearance. Why now? Well, your belly is loose—there is likely all of this extra skin and a bit of fat still kicking it right on your midsection. To squeeze that into a pair of pants is just wrong. You'll be uncomfortable and risking "the overhang." You know, when you bend

style watch: transition wear

The newest thing in maternity wear is transition wear. Some designers have added a new collection to their lines for that "fourth trimester" when we all struggle to find something to wear. Definitely something to look into, as these clothes don't even resemble maternity wear yet still have a lot of the fit your body needs while shedding those baby pounds.

over and all of that extra skin topples over the top of your jeans? *Yuck*. If you stick to loose and low, you'll be totally golden—and all nice and neatly tucked away.

★ **First Trimester Digs:** Now's the time to pull out those bigger jeans and cargos that you purchased back in the first trimester, much as it may pain you to do so. Just remember that it's only temporary. And if you need to, keep out a pair or two of those low-waisted maternity jeans for those days when there is just nothing else that'll do. Listen, Gwyneth did it and so can you!

★ **Boot Leg, Baby:** Boot-cut pants are just oh so flattering, even when you're in a postpartum rut. Look for pants in this cut to take you through this transition time—and when you get back down to your goal weight, just take them on in to your tailor.

★ **Slender Skirts:** A-line and long, romantic bohemian-inspired skirts are the best for this transitional wardrobe. They flatter even the largest frames and help conceal any extra wiggle around your derriere. Team them up with boots or sandals, a loose top, and some fun jewelry and you've got a postpartum look that simply rocks.

FROM A PRO

"I'll let you in on a little secret—a product I sell and personally swear by . . . the Rebelt panty by Anita (aka girdle) for those early postpartum weeks! I was first introduced to this product by my Italian mother-in-law, who brought me two, direct from Rome, in beautiful brocade fabric upon the birth of my first child. She told me my sister-in-law had used them and I agreed to try them and was completely convinced! They're designed to keep your tummy taut in those postpartum weeks when the uterus is healing; we usually recommend using from two weeks to six weeks postpartum. With triple rows of hooks and eyes . . . think bra hooks . . . you work your way in every few weeks. And if you're not convinced that there is any permanent benefit achieved here, I promise you . . . the instant gratification a 'taut tummy' is able to provide during what I'll only refer to as 'very hormonal weeks' is priceless!"

—KATIE TAGLIAVIA,
owner of 9 Months, key retailer

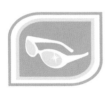

Star Secret: Britney Spears

"Once I get the okay from my doctor to start working out, I am there! My goal is to spend time with my babies and concentrate on getting my body back in shape. I love being in a disciplined workout routine and can't wait to get back on track with that." (Britney tells Rock Star Momma *that the biggest change in her body during her pregnancies is that she's not as muscular as she usually is. Sound familiar?*)

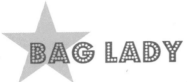

BAG LADY

Who doesn't want the *perfect* diaper bag? One that screams hip but maintains serious functionality and durability, too. For the first twelve months, it's just gotta be big. You'll end up tossing in a bunch of diapers, diaper changing pad, wipes, diaper rash cream, clothes, clothes, and more clothes, hats, socks, spit-up cloths, sunscreen, binkies, bottles, food, toys, and more. Pretty much the kitchen sink, right? So you've gotta have a bag that can handle it all, too.

Think big. Think hip. Think functional. Think sassy. Bags in metallic. Bags with bling. Bags that totally rock and look like a sling. Totes, backpacks, straps with grommets, bags with studs. Bright colors. You'll love it all—as long as it's hip, cool, *and* functional. Yes, FUNCTIONAL! It's gotta be baby *and* momma friendly. That said, here are a few rock star momma rules to remember before you head out on your quest for that bag. Check it out:

First off, anything with bunnies, fire trucks, bears, lions, sailboats, or anything else of that nature is just *not okay*. Got it? You are a hip chick. You are a MILF! You are not that girl who does teddy bears and balloons, especially not on a diaper bag, so toss out those freebie wannabe diaper bags the doctor's office and hospital gave you—they are free for a reason!!!

Second, it's got to be BIG. This bag has got to hold ALL of your baby paraphernalia, as well as your stuff.

Third, it's got to have compartments—there is nothing

"While the mechanics of the way people make and have kids hasn't changed much in hundreds of years, what we parents expect it to be has changed. Nobody wants to surrender who they are as people when they become parents. So don't compromise. Dress yourself and your kids in cool gear and keep rockin'."

—STEVE GRANVILLE,
cofounder of Fleurville

worse than trying to fish for an extra binky with one arm at the bottom of your diaper bag while holding your baby in the other. Find a bag with many compartments to help keep you superorganized—and stress-free.

Last, skip any bags that have built-in diaper changing pads that are part of the bag's framework. They are a total nightmare—they fall over and are more in the way than helpful. Rather, go for bags that have a separate roll-up diaper-changing pad inside. Plus, that way you can toss the pad in the laundry, as needed.

Finding the right bag doesn't have to be a task, honest. Think out of the box—you don't have to carry a traditional diaper bag. Thankfully, many leading designers have bags that readily double as diaper bags, which make them a great investment because when you're done with the diaper bag stage—well, if they're not TOTALLY trashed—you can still use 'em as a handy tote. (The reality of this happening is probably slim, but it's still an option if your bag can withstand a couple years of baby wear and tear!)

ROCK STAR DADDY DIAPER BAGS!

Okay, so now that you've scooped up a chic new diaper bag for yourself, why not hook up your hubby with his very own diaper bag? I've asked the creator of and the original "Diaper Dude," Chris Pegula, to help get your man a bag just as cool as the one you're rockin'!

ROCK STAR DADDY DIAPER BAGS

1. *Comfort* – Make sure you choose a bag that feels good to you. Remember, you can pull off anything if you have the confidence, but confidence will only come with comfort. It may look cool to you but you will make it look even cooler if it fits comfortably.

2. *Function* – A diaper bag can look as hip as ever, but if it's not functional don't choose it. Rock star dads are always in control. You need a bag that will assist you when you are in those times of need. Look for bags that offer quick accessibility to bottles, wipes, pacifiers, etc.

3. *Look* – Choose a bag that reflects your style. Whether you are a conservative or funky dude, there is a wide range of bags that can suit you.

4. *Durability* — What good is a diaper bag if you can only use it once or twice? Give it the ol' dad test. A tug here, a tug there. Make sure it will last. Durable fabrics like nylon and canvas are a good start. Remember, you are going to be dodging plenty of baby's recycled food from both ends (if you get my drift) so choose a durable fabric that will clean easily and will keep you looking like a star.

 Besides a diaper bag, what's the next big purchase? On the hunt for that perfect stroller? That's a whole other book! But I will leave you with this: a must-have tip from a pro about strollers . . . from the stunning Bugaboo collection (it doesn't get any better than a Bugaboo!):

"It began when I looked at strollers in the street in the early nineties, I couldn't imagine myself walking behind such ugly and nonperforming strollers. I imagined myself as an active parent, wanting to go to the mountains, the beach, into town, and continuing the lifestyle I had at that time. When you do not have children, you are not aware of all the functionalities you will be needing. You just look at how a stroller looks. As a product designer, I saw it as a huge challenge and opportunity to make a difference and come up with a stroller that would incorporate the needs of modern parents and that would increase their freedom of movement in an innovative way, and that would also look great. For modern parents, it is both design and functionality that are the most important."

—MAX BARENBRUG,
founder and CTO of Bugaboo

"It's a great time to be expecting: There are so many more options for today's modern pregnant woman. From stylish maternity clothing that can also be mixed with nonpregnancy clothing for a unique look to great skin products and exercise classes tailored to pregnant women. And for the nursery and layette, there are a surprising number of cool furniture lines, hip clothing, and strollers for new moms who want baby items that work with their lifestyles."

—SUSAN MALONEY,
founder/editor in chief of UrbanBaby.com

Now, this might be a little premature for this book, but I just had to say this. THANK the GODS above that the baby and kids marketplace is changing rapidly to deliver what modern mommas and papas want. No longer are parents limited to boring cribs and dull nursery decor. The market is ON FIRE and you will be the beneficiary of all this! Think about it . . . Pottery Barn now has a dedicated kids store!!! And I can go on and on about all the amazing, fresh designers out there that have really lit a fire in the baby and kids market. Be sure to check out all the amazing resources in the **Shopping Bag** chapter. You can thank me later!

the last word

That's it, mommas! You have done it—you've not only made it through your pregnancy, but into the world of all things postpartum panache. In the next few weeks and months, you'll see your bod return to it's pre-pregnancy bodaciousness, I promise. But give it time. Be gentle on yourself. Treat yourself kindly—remember it's not just your new baby that needs TLC. You do, too, momma. After all, you've just pulled off the biggest miracle in the world!

I've sincerely loved joining you on your journey through the crazy, sexy, fabulous world of rock star mommahood. I've just got one final promise: I'll be right here rockin' and rollin' with you next time round! See you then, rock star momma!

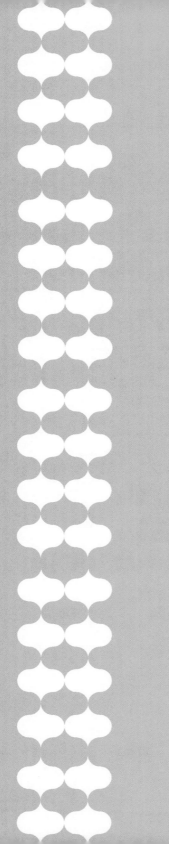

CHAPTER 9

swipe their style

Okay, so now you know everything you need to know to work it and be beautiful during your pregnancy. You have all the ammo necessary to sashay into any room during these forty wonderful weeks! You can do it, I know you can, but in case you need an added bit of encouragement, I'll leave you with these valuable tips I've learned from some of my favorite famous bellies. Here's Heidi, Gwen, Sarah, and Brooke, one last time, to help you become hip, haute, and oh so chic before you indulge in the **Shopping Bag** chapter.

The world is your catwalk, so read on and *WALK THIS WAY. . . .*

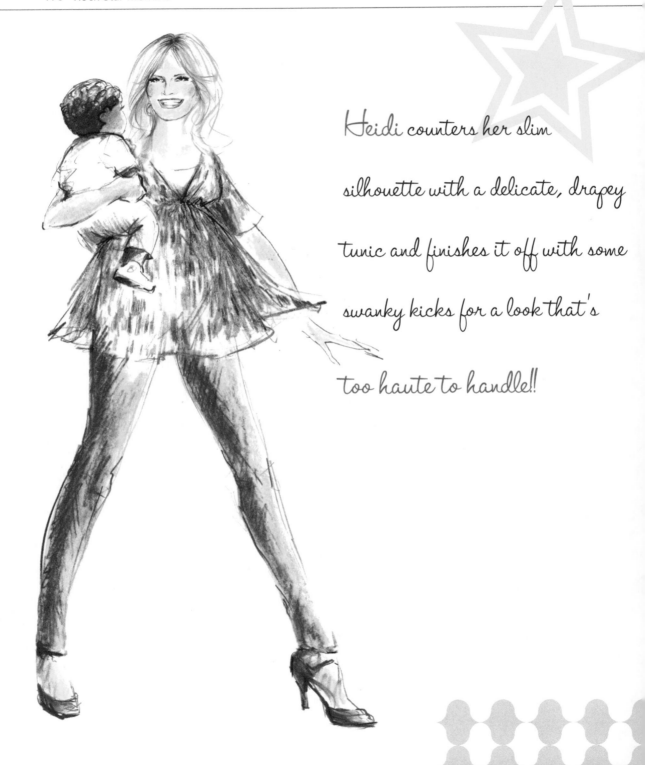

Heidi counters her slim silhouette with a delicate, drapey tunic and finishes it off with some swanky kicks for a look that's too haute to handle!!

★ *Fresh Face:* With clean, simple makeup, Heidi's natural skin radiates. Apply shimmery shadow on your brow bone and inner corners of your eyes to get a natural glow of your own.

★ *Lash, Lash Baby!:* Coat your lashes with an extra layer of mascara, focusing a bit more on the outer lashes to achieve stunning, catlike eyes. That extra touch of top-coat adds the "eye-catching" final touch!

★ *Tinted Love:* Less is more for Heidi and should be for you too on casual cool days. If you are blessed with beautiful lips, then a super shiny lip gloss with a hint of color is all you'll need for a striking smile.

★ *Think Pink:* Choose light and bright tones when searching for your perfect blush. A simple stroke on your cheeks is an effortless way to brighten your look.

★ *The Mane Event:* Casual cool hair never looked so good. For bouncy summery hair that's full of movement, apply your favorite root amplifier before blow-drying to help amplify those tresses. Then, invest in a great roller brush and blow away.

★ *Peg Leg:* Billowy blouses and tunics are back in fashion but you're going to need to pair them with skinny jeans for balance. And be sure that those skinny's are long and lean. No high-waters here!

And, as you may already know or are about to find out, to complete the look is the world's best "accessory" in tow—your precious baby!

Heidi Klum

★ *"Hollaback Girl"*: W-O-W! Gwen creates a most modern version of the classic 1950s cream lipsticks. Simply glamorous velvety red lips are just perfect for your red-carpet couture look. *No better lip service than this!*

★ *"Just a Girl"*: Accessorize in style with metallic gold bangles. The more the merrier since these should be your only accessories with a dress this fierce!

★ *"Rock Steady"*: Heavy black eyeliner presents well-defined eyes and sets the tone for this nighttime-nice look. Accent with shimmery metallic shadow shades to complete your diva-licious look.

★ *"Wind It Up"*: Consistent with so much of Gwen's style, her famous bright-white tresses manage to simultaneously call to mind old-school Hollywood with modern-day punk. Pulled back with a look that's definitely Gwen and most definitely seductive, this look can bring your hair from the red carpet to reality.

★ *"Hey Baby"*: The empire line in this ravishing design allows you to flaunt and flatter that gorgeous belly you're rockin'!

★ *"Hella Good"*: With an animal instinct we all know and love, Gwen allows the leopard print to simply speak for itself. *Enough said…*

All the glamour and style-talk aside, remind yourself that true beauty lies "Underneath It All."

Gwen Stefani

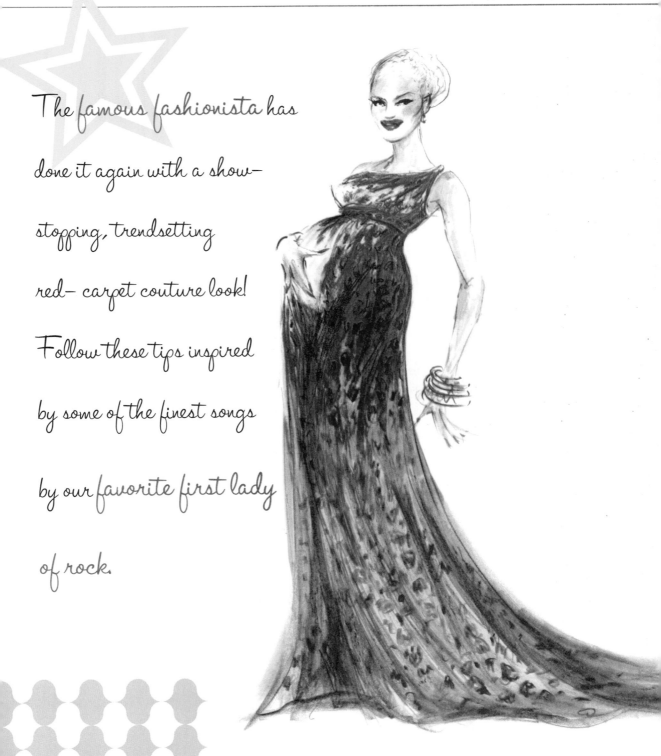

The famous fashionista has done it again with a show-stopping, trendsetting red-carpet couture look! Follow these tips inspired by some of the finest songs by our favorite first lady of rock.

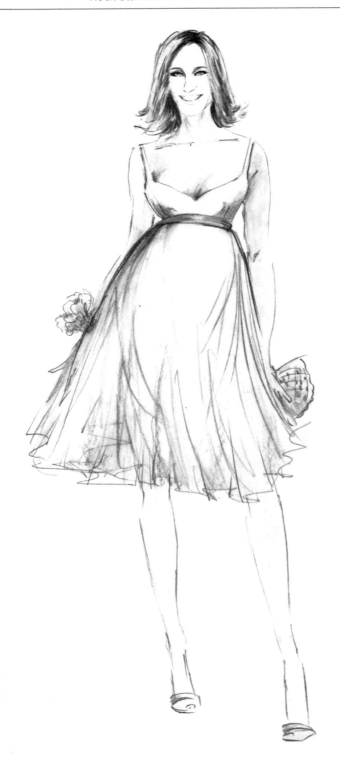

For years,

Sarah Jessica Parker

has been admired as a fashion

icon. Always known for her

progressive sense of style,

whether expecting or not, this

lady is the mother of all

haute couture.

★ *Dress to Impress*: A little flowy dress with a loosely cut silhouette looks best when worn above the knee with a sweet, sexy heel.

★ *Bright Eyes*: Add depth and definition to your eyes with a creamy eyeliner crayon (I love the new wider pencil versions!). Search for metallic shades that contain a hint of sparkling glitter particles that reflect the light for a most glamorous finish.

★ *In Small Packages*: A subtle, feminine clutch in a contrasting color is small on size yet big on style. Look for structured shapes with jeweled clasps or rounded lines with simple adornments.

★ *Less Is More*: Yep, I said it. . . . Sarah Jessica Parker lets this dress speak for itself. No need to overdo this look. A clean neck simply draws attention to the stunning dress and Sarah's flawless bod!

★ *Flower Power*: The simple yet sweet added touch of a wintery-white flower wrapped around your wrist rounds out this smart and elegant look.

★ *Fancy Footwork*: Go city chic with a strappy stiletto in metallic silver or gold. A delicate heel also gives the illusion of endlessly long legs…*so flattering!*

What would Carrie Bradshaw think?

Sarah Jessica Parker

★ *Momma's Got a Brand New Bag:* Big is *back!* The bottomless bag has taken on a most compelling cosmopolitan quality. Look for bags in buttery-soft, supple leathers, and tried-and-true shapes. I also love those that are hardware-free for a completely unique and sleek look.

★ *Skin Is In!:* Got a great belly? Show it off in a sweet, subtle fashion. With a track jacket that barely covers your burgeoning belly combined with low-rider drawstring trackpants, your belly has arrived!

★ *Too Cool Tracksuit:* Velvety-soft cotton velour not only feels good but looks amazing! Under-the-belly cuts are always best. Look for styles with an adjustable drawstring for those last few weeks when you'll need all the extra room you can get!

★ *Head Gear:* Be casual cool with a bucket hat atop natural, clean messy hair. Effortlessly chic!

★ *Walk This Way:* Popularized by the uberchic Audrey Hepburn, the kitten heel is a perfect option for casual cool days. Opt to pair these with your tracksuit rather than your seen-better-days tennis shoes for a simply stylish look.

★ *Polished Glow:* Let your inner glow shine through with simple, trouble-free makeup. I love the new blush sticks that give cheeks (and lips too!) that barely-there, fresh-faced look. Uncomplicated and easy to apply, these give you a gorgeous glow and finish, making your skin flawless in no time at all!

Brooke Shields

Brooke Shields has managed to maintain that fabulous natural beauty throughout her life. She's graced our presence for nearly two decades with those sultry eyes, sexy hair, and long legs. It's no wonder she's America's sweetheart!

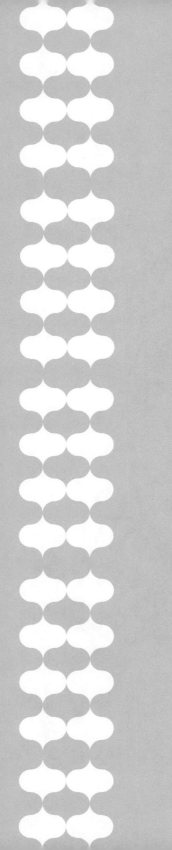

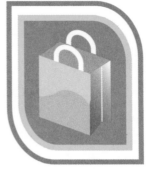

CHAPTER 10

SHOPPING BAG

★ ★

Nobody loves shopping more than I do, and as I've promised throughout the book, this last chapter is chock-full of resources for you to find everything you just read about, and then some. I've spent years finding the very best products, websites, books, clothes, accessories, and more, and now I would love to share them with you. You can always check out www.rockstarmomma.com for the very latest products, trends, and stores that were yet to be conceived when this baby went to print.

dot coms for hot moms

▬▬▬ General pregnancy resource websites

★ www.babycenter.com

★ www.babyzone.com

★ www.pregnancyandbaby.com

★ www.pregnancydaily.com

★ www.pregnancystore.com

★ www.pregnancytoday.com

★ www.askdrsears.com   the well-known doctor and author Dr. Sears

★ www.parenthood.com

★ www.iparenting.com   mothering resource

★ www.ivillage.com

★ www.mothercare.com

★ www.allaboutmoms.com

★ www.mommyhelp.com

★ www.sheknows.com   I go to the Pregnancy and Baby sections for
                              endless information

Overall health / medical / well-being resource websites

★ www.abog.org — American Board of Obstetrics & Gynecology

★ www.acog.org — American College of Obstetricians & Gynecologists

★ www.aap.com — American Academy of Pediatrics

★ www.aafp.org — American Academy of Family Physicians

★ www.visembryo.com — comprehensive resource for info on human development

★ www.lamaze.org — locate a Lamaze class

★ www.lamaze-childbirth.com —

★ www.doulanetwork.com — locate a doula in your area

★ www.dona.org — Doulas of North America

★ www.midwifeinfo.com — locate a midwife

★ www.otispregnancy.org — medical resource

★ www.4women.gov — pregnancy health/nutrition

★ www.eatright.org — nutritional information

★ www.babyfit.com — pregnancy fitness

★ www.maternalfitness.com prenatal/postpartum exercise and more

★ www.yogabirth.com yoga site for the expecting

★ www.bradleybirth.com The Bradley Method/childbirth education

★ www.icea.com International Childbirth Education Organization

★ www.childbirthclasstogo.com

★ www.childbirthconnection.org

★ www.birthingbetter.com

★ www.plus-size-pregnancy.org

★ www.cordblood.com cord blood banking—*research this very important topic!!*

★ www.cryo-cell.com cord blood banking

★ www.maternitywise.org national program to provide evidence-based maternity care

Consumer safety information resource websites

★ www.consumerreports.org

★ www.consumer.gov/children.htm

★ www.jpma.org   Juvenile Products Manufacturers Association

★ www.cpsc.gov   Consumer Products Safety Commission

★ www.childproductsafety.com

★ www.ewg.org/reports/skindeep2

★ www.ibabyproof.com   complete baby-proofing and safety website

★ www.safeandsecurebaby.com everything for making your home a safe place
                                 for your new baby

★ www.safebeginnings.com   more childproofing products and home safety
                                 items

Breast-feeding resource websites

★ www.lalecheleague.org

★ www.medela.com

★ www.pumpstation.com

★ www.awomanswork.com

★ www.motherwear.com

★ www.gotmom.org

★ www.nursingbaby.com

Haute momma: maternity fashion websites

★ www.childishclothing.com

★ www.apeainthepod.com

Britney Spears tells me this is her favorite maternity store. "Their clothes just fit so perfectly and it's not the traditional maternity wear. All of their clothes are so stylish!"

★ www.babystyle.com

★ www.nordstrom.com

★ www.neimanmarcus.com

★ www.topshop.com

★ www.bellydancematernity.com

★ www.duematernity.com

★ www.picklesandicecream.com

★ www.lizlange.com

★ www.japaneseweekend.com

★ www.cadeaumaternity.com

★ www.meetmeinmiami.com

★ www.olianmaternity.com

★ www.julietdream.com

★ www.laurenkiyomi.com

★ www.gap.com

★ www.target.com

★ www.shopbop.com

★ www.9monthsinc.com

★ www.chiarakruza.com

★ www.elinotto.com

★ www.bellyliciousmaternity.com

★ www.momstheword.com

★ www.majamas.com

★ www.bellablumaternity.com

★ www.tummiesmaternity.com

★ www.evalillian.com

★ www.maternnity.ca   great Canadian website with fashion and more

★ www.cheekymonkey.ca   another great Canadian website for pregnant
                             women

★ www.9london.co.uk — chic London maternity boutique and fabulous website

★ www.bloomingmarvellous.co.uk — great quality maternity wear based out of the UK and a great overall website

★ www.blossommotherandchild.com — *gorgeous* maternity wear from *top* runway designers—*get ready to spend some $$$*

★ www.bumpsville.com — funky, stylish, high-end UK maternity store/website

★ www.dorothyperkins.co.uk — multiple locations around the UK—good casual maternity selection

★ www.eliasandgrace.com — located in London (a Gwen Stefani favorite)—offers a modern and versatile approach to everything maternity

★ www.formes.com — UK—high quality maternity fashion

★ www.laconception.co.uk — another quality, stylish site and store in London

★ www.pushmaternity.com — UK store/website—very fashionable!

★ www.mamasandpapas.com — UK designer maternity/fashion website

★ www.funmum.com — UK fashion maternity wear

★ www.cravematernity.co.uk — UK maternity clothes and wear

★ www.isabellaoliver.com — small but chic UK collection

★ www.avenue-des-bebes.com   French maternity line

★ www.vertbaudet.co.uk   French fashion for mommas and kids

★ www.rubyvan.com   ultrahip tees and tanks for the hip momma-to-be

★ www.mothersinmotion.com   maternity exercise clothing

★ www.fitmaternity.com   comfortable maternity activewear

★ www.yogabirth.com   yoga attire for the expecting

★ www.sleepyheads.com   remember the cool pjs I was talking about?

★ www.pajamagram.com   check out the section for new moms

★ www.ellemacphersonintimates.com

★ www.condessainc.com   "breast-feeding lingerie"—*gorgeous!*

★ www.bellamaterna.com   amazing maternity and nursing bras and so much more!

★ www.bravadodesigns.com   breast-feeding bras

★ www.awomanswork.com   maternity and breast-feeding wear

★ www.figleaves.com   online lingerie store with a maternity department

★ www.spanx.com   Spanx maternity pantyhose and new nursing bras

★ www.mothernaturebras.co.uk   online store, located in the UK—great bras!

★ www.royce-lingerie.co.uk   UK—stylish wire-free nursing/maternity bras

★ www.momsnightout.com   elegant formal wear for pregnant women

Beauty-licious websites

★ www.sephora.com

★ www.saffronrouge.com   Sells only products made with certified organic ingredients wherever possible. All their products are plant and/or mineral based, 100 percent natural, and free of synthetic chemicals, preservatives, fragrances, and colors, and not tested on animals. They also disclose all ingredients for every item they sell.

★ www.beautyhabit.com   great beauty site that stocks the best beauty brands for expecting moms and new babies

★ www.theorganicpharmacy.com   gorgeous site dedicated to health and beauty using organic products

★ www.edamamespa.com   maternity spa/website by Destination Maternity

★ www.gloss.com   you can never have enough lip gloss!

★ www.jaquabeauty.com   home of the famous "super-sweet" beauty products

★ www.mamamio.com   A one-stop shop! I *love* this site!

★ www.bellamama.com   Another one-stop shop! Great gift sets too!

★ www.erbaviva.com   all-natural, organic skin-care products for
                             momma-to-be and baby

★ www.mustela.com   *the* essential skin-care line for momma-to-be
                             and baby

★ www.bellicosmetics.com   you really should check out their Anti-Chloasma
                             Facial Sunscreen SPF 25 and Pure Comfort
                             Nipple Cream.

★ www.basqnyc.com   They have the highest-quality pregnancy skin
                             care available. Note:Heidi Klum is a fan.

★ www.motherlove.com   a full collection of herbal products made just for
                             pregnant gals

★ www.pharmacopia.net   check out the Lavender Body Oil with Roman
                             Chamomile (I recommend using in the second
                             and third trimesters to combat headaches,
                             aches, and pains)

★ www.ensantlotions.com   Skin-care line dedicated to pregnant women
                             and the changes their bodies endure both
                             during and after pregnancy. Check out the Peri
                             Balm to help minimize perineal tearing.

★ www.mothersintuition.com   home of the famous Tummy Honey Butter-
                             Stretch Mark Prevention Butter

★ www.apivita.com   you will love the Apivita Propoline product line
                             (all natural)

★ www.kiehls.com

★ www.motherearthandbaby.com

★ www.aroma1.com   see Maternity and Baby section

★ www.nealsyardremedies.com   see Mother and Baby section

★ www.californiababy.com

★ www.babybearshop.com

★ www.mdmoms.com

★ www.avalonorganics.com

★ www.amazon.com   they carry the Modelco Cool Feet Airbrush Catwalk Heels spray that I was telling you about!

★ www.blissbymom.com

★ www.palmerscocoabutter.com   check out their Mother and Baby section

★ www.labelladonna.com   a full line of mineral-based cosmetics

★ www.janeiredale.com   another great line of mineral-based cosmetics

★ www.bareescentuals.com   mineral-based cosmetics

★ www.mineralogie.biz   mineral-based cosmetics

★ www.colorescience.com   mineral-based cosmetics

★ www.barefootandpregnant.com

Shout it out: announcements/invites/paper goods websites

★ www.soolip.com

★ www.shopiomoi.com

★ www.chelseapaper.com

★ www.sugarpaper.com

★ www.babyidesign.com

★ www.rockpaperscissors.com

★ www.groovypaper.com

★ www.storkavenue.com

★ www.jellyandanchovy.com

★ www.paperinkstudio.com

★ www.shwamy.com

★ www.smythson.com   only the finest paper and a celeb favorite—very pricey!

★ www.tinyprints.com

★ www.joybymellim.com

★ www.einvite.com

★ www.papercupdesign.com

★ www.tinaj.com

★ www.laurengdesigns.com

★ www.felixdoolittle.com   these are tiny watercolors/full illustrations—so different from your typical invite or announcement—with rounded corners and complementing illustrated envelopes (unique and gorgeous!)

★ www.oplusd.com   sassy and obnoxiously honest, but *so* clever!

★ www.pearlpapers.com

★ www.elumdesigns.com

★ www.mangoink.com   So clever! Uses your own photography and text for a most unique announcement or invite.

★ www.pbkisses   modern stationery

★ www.fabulousstationery.com

★ www.bumblebeepress.com

★ www.ediblesinc.com   greeting card/announcement *cookie!*

★ www.elenis.com   check out the "Special Delivery Girl" and "Bundle of Boy" items

★ www.photo.stamps.com   put your baby's picture on a photo stamp!

MODERN NURSERY MUST-HAVES WEBSITES

★ www.babygeared.com

★ www.modernseed.com

★ www.egiggle.com

★ www.geniusjones.com

★ www.modernnursery.com

★ www.zacandzoe.com

★ www.moderntots.com

★ www.modernmini.com

★ www.sparkability.com

★ www.mimmobaby.com

★ www.babystyle.com

★ www.landofnod.com

★ www.poshtots.com   over-the-top designer nursery furniture and accessories

★ www.nettocollection.com   David Netto Nursery furniture and accessories

★ www.kuhl-linscomb.com

★ www.yoyashop.com

★ www.piccolinionline.com — hip Los Angeles store enters cyberspace

★ www.petittresor.com — the ultrahip Beverly Hills baby boutique frequented by Hollywood's biggest celebs!

★ www.ducducnyc.com

★ www.celeryfurniture.com — LOVE this line of nursery room furniture! So chic!

★ www.oeufnyc.com

★ www.nurseryworks.net

★ www.ooba.com

★ www.argington.com

★ www.wendybellissimo.com — her line is now carried exclusively at Babies "R" Us

★ www.miguelonline.com — unique variety of cribs all handmade in Italy

★ www.lazarsfurniture.com — hip Chicago store

★ www.lrstudiofurniture.com — Laura Rittenhouse crib in mahogany and sterling silver! Yep, and it's 5K but worth every penny if you can afford it! Moon and stars silver inlays on sides make this an heirloom piece you will forever admire! This elegant crib can also be custom designed with an original design.

★ www.koolroomz.net

★ www.cradleandcrayon.com

★ www.artbebe.com   cool room decor and more site

★ www.purbebe.com   eco-friendly baby boutique, organic cotton
                                     baby clothes and natural baby products

★ www.propertyfurniture.com

★ www.designpublic.com   fresh new designs for families

★ www.cocoacrayon.com

★ www.pokkadots.com

★ www.smallconcept.com

★ www.2modern.com

★ www.modernkid.com   extensive selection of modern nursery good-
                                     ies—Canadian store

★ www.forestandzoe   designer duds for babies and more

★ www.oompa.com

★ www.citysprouts.com

★ www.ikea.com   but it might be better to go to the stores to see
                                     in person if you can

★ www.walmart.com   Who would have ever thought Wal-Mart could
                                     be design-savvy and cool! I just love their new
                                     Modern Nursery Collection!

★ www.potterybarnkids.com

★ www.edgemodern.com — check out the latest Dwell bedding

★ www.petuniapetunia.com — I love the crib bedding and blankets!

★ www.kukunest.com — *adorable* bedding!

★ www.serenaandlily.com — classic, beautiful bedding

★ www.gustavmaxwell.com — modern bedding and accessories

★ www.flor.com — amazing floor covering

★ www.brightoctober.com — modern online boutique for children/unique assortment of European toys

★ www.adriftmobiles.com — gorgeous mobiles for your nursery, hand-crafted in San Francisco

★ www.grahambrown.com — check out their paintable wallpaper for kids, called "Frames" by Taylor and Wood—never too early to get those walls ready for crayons!

★ www.velocityartanddesign.com — check out the Playtime Wallpapers by London-based design studio Absolute Zero Degrees

★ www.avalisa.com — bold wall decor for your baby's room

★ www.whatisblik.com — adorable wall decals!

★ www.shannonlowry.com — limited-edition artwork for your nursery

★ www.weegallery.com — the name says it all—artwork for little ones!

★ www.tobiwooddesigns.com — simple yet beautiful wall art for your nursery

★ www.strawberryluna.com — For the real rock star baby! Try these rock posters in your little one's room, rather than trains and butterflies!

★ www.babyohmy.com — natural and eco-friendly gifts for modern and design-savvy parents

★ www.oliebollen.com

★ www.babyant.com — multifaceted retailer with so much to offer and good for basics

★ www.babybecause.com

★ www.geniusbabies.com — infant toys and enrichment products

★ www.mbeans.com — baby gear, toys, surprises, newsletter—overall cool site for hip parents!

★ www.distinctivenurseries.com

★ www.classymommy.com — gifts for mom and baby and more

★ www.sozousa.com

★ www.henryandlulu.com

★ www.nova68.com

★ www.tinytruffles.com

★ www.thebabyjoint.com

★ www.babybrowns.com

★ www.livingincomfort.com

★ www.maukilo.com

★ www.dandelionbaby.com   adorable little kids' stuff

★ www.littlebits.com   for those adorable car seat covers and much, much more!

★ www.babybeddingtown.com   just as the name suggests—a lot to look at on this site . . . could be overwhelming!

Modern Baby Gear Websites

★ www.fleurville.com

★ www.bugaboo.com

★ www.orbitbaby.com   revolutionary new baby car seat and stroller (modular system)

★ www.stokke.com   ubercool stroller in rad colors!

★ www.bumbleride.com   gorgeous strollers!

★ www.maclarenbaby.com

★ www.uppababy.com   I just love the Vista stroller system

★ www.tinyride.com   specialty retailer of baby strollers, joggers, and car seats

★ www.svanusa.com   the hippest bouncer in town!

★ www.elitecarseats.com   carries the best in full range of car seats

★ www.kolcraft.com   I love (and so will you!) their car seat carrier stroller

★ www.diaperdude.com   specializes in diaper bags for men

★ www.skiphop.com

★ www.dantebeatrix.com

★ www.petuniapicklebottom.com

★ www.diaperbags.com   *huge*, quality selection of bags in all styles

★ www.chesterhandbags.com

★ www.miabossi.com

★ www.littlebits.com   remember those car-seat covers I mentioned by Monica Rodgers!

★ www.jjcoleusa.com

★ www.babybjorn.com

★ www.billamberg.com   check out the papoose for babies and more

★ www.happybabyproducts.com   check out the MobiCam Baby Monitor, winner of the *Wall Street Journal*'s 2005 monitor review

★ www.gracobaby.com

★ www.infantino.com

★ www.aventamerica.com

★ www.mamasandpapas.co.uk   look for the ZIKO Frankie Stroller—Gwen Stefani's got one in metallic *gold!*

★ www.tinydodo.com   amazing design ideas and much more for babies (Dutch store but ships international)

Blogs you should know about

★ www.urbanbaby.com

★ www.dailycandykids.com

★ www.coochicoos.com   great baby design/product blog for modern parents

★ www.weecitizens.com

★ www.nonchalantmom.com   just plain cool online store and resource site for modern parents

★ www.cookiemag.com/magazine/blogs/daysitter   blog for *Cookie* magazine

★ www.daddydrama.com

★ www.modernmom.com

★ www.designmom.com   cool blog for design moms

★ www.celebrity-babies.com

★ www.babygadget.net

★ www.babble.com   online community for hip urban parents

★ www.coolmompicks.com

★ www.mothersclick.com

★ www.mommytrackd.com   great site geared toward working mothers

★ www.justmommies.com

★ www.parenthacks.com

★ www.beforebaby.com

★ www.thefunkystork.com   blog site and more for modern expectant fathers

★ www.5minutesformom.com   blogging, shopping, parenting

★ www.brandnewmom.com

Baby shower resource websites

★ www.babyshower101.com

★ www.baby-shower.com

★ www.babyshowercentral.com

★ www.babyshowergamesatoz.com

★ www.babybingo.com

★ www.thebabyshowersite.com

★ www.abcfavors.com

★ www.ababyshower.com

★ www.plumparty.com

★ www.welcomebaby.com

Name-DROPPING OR THE NAME GAME: BABY NAME WEBSITES

★ www.babynamer.com

★ www.babynames.com

★ www.babynamesworld.com   meaning and place of origin

★ www.babychatter.com   popularity, meaning, origin

★ www.popularbabynames.com

★ www.babynameguide.com   offers search by category

★ www.zoope.com

★ www.babynameaddicts.com

★ www.babynamemachine.com

★ www.babynology.com

★ www.babynamecorner.com

★ www.thenamemachine.com

★ www.babynamewizard.com

★ www.cool-baby-names.com

★ www.babynamenetwork.com

★ www.123-baby-names.com

★ www.babynameguide.com

★ www.babynameorigins.com

read all about it

Books and magazines you should definitely check out!

Magazines

★ *Fit Pregnancy*

★ *Cookie*

★ *Parents*

★ *Parenting*

★ *Child*

★ *American Baby*

★ *Baby Talk*

★ *Pregnancy*

★ *Junior (UK import)*

★ *Baby Couture*

▰▰ Books

★ *The Girlfriends' Guide to Pregnancy* by Vicki Iovine

★ *The Pregnancy Book* by William Sears

★ *The Birth Book* by William Sears

★ *The Breastfeeding Book* by Martha and William Sears

★ *The Baby Book* by William Sears

★ *What to Expect When You're Expecting* by Heidi Murkoff

★ *From Here to Maternity: The Education of a Rookie Mom* by Beth Teitell

★ *Mayo Clinic Complete Book of Pregnancy & Baby's First Year* by Mayo Clinic/ William Morrow

★ *The Glow: The Journey to Motherhood* by Danica Perez (photography book)

★ *What to Eat When You're Expecting* by Arlene Eisenberg

★ *Eating for Pregnancy: An Essential Guide to Nutrition with Recipes for the Whole Family* by Catherine Jones and Rose Ann Hudson

★ *The Expectant Father: Facts, Tips, and Advice for Dads-to-Be* by Armin A. Brott

★ *My Boys Can Swim: The Official Guy's Guide to Pregnancy* by Ian Davis

★ *A Child Is Born* by Lennart Nilsson

★ *Birthing from Within: An Extra-Ordinary Guide to Childbirth Preparation* by Pam England and Rob Horowitz

★ *The Birth That's Right for You: A Doctor and a Doula Help You Choose and Customize the Best Birth Option to Fit Your Needs* by Amen Ness, M.D., Lisa Gould Rubin, C.D., C.C.E., and Jackie Frederick-Berner

★ *Wendy Bellissimo Nesting* by Wendy Bellissimo and Leslie Lehr Spirson (comes with a DVD and features over fifty nurseries—great design inspiration and help!)

★ *The Ninth Month* by Catherine Steinmann (photography book)

★ *Miracle: A Celebration of New Life* by Anne Geddes and Celine Dion

★ *Pure* by Anne Geddes (photography book)

★ *The Baby Owner's Manual* by Louis Borgenicht, M.D., and Joe Borgenicht, D.A.D.

★ *The Diaper Diaries: The Poop on the First Year of Motherhood* by Cynthia L. Copeland

★ *Crib Notes: A Random Reference for the Modern Parent* by Amy Maniatis and Elizabeth Weil

★ *How to Make a Pregnant Woman Happy* by Uzzi Reiss, M.D., OB/GYN, and Yfat M. Reiss

★ *The Lila Guide: Baby Gear Buyer's Guide 2005*

★ *The Purple Book Baby: Baby and Maternity Edition* by Hillary Mendelsohn

★ *20,001 Names for Baby: Revised and Updated* by Carol McD. Wallace

music to momma's ears: cds

★ *Baby Einstein* (lullaby classics)

★ *Mozart for Mothers-to-Be*

★ *Ultra Sound: Music for the Unborn Child* by Claude Debussy

★ *Tune Your Brain: Pregnancy and Childbirth*

★ *Pregnancy Relaxation: A Guide to Peaceful Beginnings* by Dana Schardt

★ *Bedtime with the Beatles: Instrumental Versions of Classic Beatles Songs*

★ *Build Your Baby's Brain*

★ *Bach for Babies: Fun and Games for Budding Brains*

★ *Mozart's Prodigy: Music for Babies and Mothers to Be*

★ *Disney Baby Lullaby: Favorite Sleepytime Songs for Baby and You*

★ *Lullaby: A Collection*

★ *Planet Sleeps* (lullabies from across the world)

★ *Golden Slumbers: A Father's Lullaby* (various jazz musicians)

★ Thievery Corporation CDs

★ Zero 7 CDs

★ The American Analog Set CDs

★ Sade CDs

. . . but nothing can replace the beautiful voice of a mom or dad

splurges and other fun things i just had to mention!

★ www.thelaboroflove.com — just for fun, you have to try the Chinese Lunar Calendar (a fun thing that just might predict the gender of your baby)

★ www.babygendermentor.com — home DNA gender testing kit—as early as five weeks after conception—200 percent money-back guarantee!

★ www.expectingmodels.com — Modeling agency dedicated only to pregnant women. If you've got it, flaunt it!

★ www.tiny-baubles.com — They have the Waiting Band. A great gift for expecting mom—an open-ended sterling silver ring with engraved messages inside—just perfect for when your wedding band won't fit anymore!

★ www.polkadotwhale.com — Baby Love Letters by Canopy Cards. Adorable cards/paper for expecting parents to write letters to their unborn baby.

★ www.babybeat.com — you can buy or rent fetal heartbeat monitors here

★ www.morningsicknesshelp.com — A site dedicated to morning sickness. Great products and support for women who suffer from the dreaded morning sickness.

★ www.threelollies.com — look for Preggie Pops—provides all-natural relief from morning sickness!

★ www.boppy.com — look for the Pregnancy Wedge, to help with those sleepness nights

★ www.onestopbaby.com — check out the pregnancy and maternity pillows

★ www.healthandyoga.com — they carry lots of great products for your well-being, including pregnancy pillows, books, and beauty products

★ www.pelvicbelt.com — I really love their pelvic belt, which reduces uncomfortable pelvic pain during pregnancy

acknowledgments

A real rock star momma knows that life is only made possible by the unconditional love of both family and friends.

Mark . . . my gorgeous husband and best friend. You are my world and everything that makes life so extraordinary. I thank you for being so supportive and easy to love.

Jack . . . my son and light of my life. I never knew life could be so miraculous. You make me proud, you make me smile, and you make our lives so complete.

Mom and Dad . . . I am who I am because of you. Thank you for teaching me everything I ever needed to know. And most important, I thank you for always being there for my family.

Susan Raihofer . . . the absolute best agent in this biz! Thank you for putting up with years of exciting chaos! This book could not have been done without you.

Greer Hendricks . . . my editor and so much more! Thank you for the guidance, the encouragement, and most of all for believing in this book. You are an amazing woman and yes, I really think you are a rock star momma!

Mandi Norwood . . . thank you for all your good advice and for such invaluable words of wisdom.

Gwyneth Paltrow . . . I cannot thank you enough for everything you have done for me. You are beautiful both inside and out and you are an inspiration for women everywhere. No other woman embodies rock star momma more than you.

Mariska Hargitay . . . thank you for making me look so good. You're an extraordinary woman and I am blessed to call you my friend.

Britney Spears . . . thank you for your fashionable contribution to this special book. You really are a rock star momma!

Joely Fisher . . . you're just too cool, I can't say enough about how rad I think you are. I'm so honored to have you as my friend.

Elle Macpherson, Jennie Garth, Kimora Lee Simmons, and T-Boz . . . thank you for your time and invaluable contributions to *Rock Star Momma*. Mommas everywhere will thank you.

Summer . . . thank you for being such a loving and loyal sister. I truly think you are a phenomenal mom.

My mother-in-law, Kerry, for always, and I mean *always*, being so darn excited about everything I do. Your belief and endless encouragement are worth more than you will ever know. Glenn, you rock, too!

Michele Dix . . . my dearest friend of all. You gave me confidence that allowed me to succeed in business and in life. You taught me about charisma and character in an industry that's known to lack both, and our friendship means the world to me. You are an incredible woman.

Jennifer Sbranti . . . a graphic design genius! Thank you for always making my ideas look so beautiful. More important, thank you for the many years of friendship.

The following people are the real experts and have created/designed/marketed the most incredible products on the market . . . and I am lucky to call them my friends and my mentors. Without their wisdom and advice, *Rock Star Momma* would not exist . . . Steve Granville (Fleurville), Kari Boiler and Max Barenbrug (Bugaboo), Susan Maloney (UrbanBaby), Sara Blakely (Spanx), Laurie McCartney (babystyle), Kathryn McRitchie (*Fit Pregnancy*), Katie Tagliavia (9 Months), Shannon DiPadova (Due Maternity), Song Pardue (Pickles and Ice Cream), Jennifer Noonan (NOM-Naissance Maternity), Debbie Ohanian (Meet Me in Miami), Dr. Katie Rodan and Dr. Fields (Rodan + Fields), Anne Diamond (Bella Materna), Paulina Quintana, Emily Meyer (Tea Collection), Annette Rubin (Belli Cosmetics), Kelli and Lauren (Basq), Wanda Wen (Soolip), Irene and Matthew (iomoi), Germaine Caprio (Majamas), Chris Pegula (Diaper

Dude), Julia Beck, Arika Chan (Arika C. Jewelry), Julie Tyler, RN, and Nicole Benoist.

Sasha Gelbart and his badass wife, Suzanne—Sasha, how you made me look that good, I will never know.

Adrienne Armstrong . . . you will never know how special your advice and love was to me during my pregnancy. Thank you for being so kind and supportive.

And to all you gorgeous bellies out there that continue to inspire me every single day, I thank you for procreating and, more important, for creating miracles called life.

—Skye

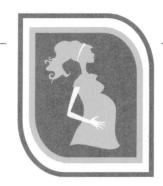

index

about the author

Skye Hoppus is the founder and owner of Childish Clothing, the ultrahip maternity and children's clothing line. She is an accomplished designer whose clothes have dressed celebrity mommas and babes and graced the pages of major magazines. Wife to Mark Hoppus of blink-182 and +44 fame, Skye knows what it means to be a rock star momma. Prior to launching Childish, Skye graduated from Pepperdine University and headed the MTV West Coast music office for nearly a decade. She lives in Los Angeles with her husband and their four-year-old son.